Beyon
the
Prescrip

Beyond the Prescription

A Doctor's Guide to Taking Charge of Your Health

LUCY McBRIDE, MD

SIMON ELEMENT

New York Amsterdam/Antwerp London
Toronto Sydney/Melbourne New Delhi

SIMON ELEMENT

An Imprint of Simon & Schuster, LLC
1230 Avenue of the Americas
New York, NY 10020

First Simon Element hardcover edition August 2026

Interior design by Janet Evans-Scanlon

Manufactured in the United States of America

10 9 8 7 6 5 4 3 2 1

Library of Congress Control Number: 2025945925

ISBN 978-1-6680-2438-6
ISBN 978-1-6680-2440-9 (ebook)

For Thad—you are my rock, my heart, my hero

CONTENTS

FOREWORD

When I first read *Beyond the Prescription*, I recognized something I've been fighting for throughout my career. Patients deserve a better framework for understanding their own bodies and a clearer vocabulary for speaking up in the doctor's office.

Dr. Lucy McBride has written the book I wish I could hand to every patient who has ever felt dismissed, confused, or overwhelmed by our healthcare system. As someone who has spent years advocating for women navigating menopause, often dismissed by a medical establishment that wasn't trained to see them, I know what happens when patients learn to become their own advocates.

What makes this book distinctive is its dual approach. First, Dr. McBride refuses to accept false binaries. She doesn't ask you to choose between conventional medicine and wellness culture, between medication and lifestyle changes, or between accepting your body and working to improve it. Instead, she offers a comprehensive framework for understanding health as an interconnected ecosystem with four quadrants: INFORMATICS, INPUTS, INFRASTRUCTURE, and INSIGHT. This framework acknowledges that your lab values don't exist in isolation from your stress levels, that your diet affects your mood as much as your cholesterol, and that your mental health is as medically relevant as your blood pressure.

Second is the book's respect for patient autonomy. Dr. McBride does not dictate decisions. She teaches you how to think about your health. She gives you the language to express what matters, the tools to interpret signals from your body, and the confidence to ask your healthcare team for the support you deserve.

My own career has centered on ensuring that patients receive evidence-based guidance delivered with compassion and clarity. Dr. McBride brings these same values to her work. She draws on decades of clinical experience without losing sight of the humanity at the heart of medicine. She acknowledges the gaps in our system while offering practical strategies to navigate them. She is honest about what medicine can deliver and equally honest about what must come from within, empowering readers to participate fully in their health journey.

The healthcare landscape is shifting. Patients are demanding more comprehensive, relationship-centered care and refusing to be treated as collections of symptoms rather than whole human beings. This book both reflects that shift and accelerates it. Every empowered patient who learns to navigate their health ecosystem becomes an advocate for better healthcare, not just for themselves, but also for everyone around them.

Dr. McBride has created a practical, scientifically grounded guide to reclaiming your health. Whether you're managing chronic conditions, navigating a fragmented healthcare system, or simply trying to understand what "health" really means for you, this book will change how you approach your body, your doctors, and your own role in your well-being.

Mary Claire Haver, MD
Author of *The New Menopause*

INTRODUCTION

Are You Okay?

"Just so we're clear, I'm only here because of my sister-in-law," Kate said, her arms folded tightly across her chest. "I've pretty much given up on traditional medicine." I set aside my laptop and asked why she'd lost faith in our system. Her answer? She had watched her father suffer through aggressive cancer treatment up until the day he died. "The last thing my dad told me was that he wished he'd just gone fishing instead."

Kate's own medical encounters had been equally frustrating: dismissive doctors who had lectured her on weight loss and whose rushed appointments ended with a prescription for medications but no specific guidance on lifestyle changes she could make to manage her diabetes and weight issues. She wasn't *against* medications; she just knew that there was more to metabolic health than prescription pills and shots. So she did what people do when they feel unheard: She started doing her own research. She tried intermittent fasting, the keto diet, and cold plunges. She listened to online influencers such as Jillian Michaels and Andrew Huberman, who seemed to speak directly to her.

Yet despite following online protocols for eighteen months, her diabetes was worse. She gained weight and felt like a failure. Kate was caught between two worlds: a medical system that treated her like a number on a scale and a wellness culture that promised better health through willpower alone.

"I completely understand your frustration," I told her.

My patient Linda had a different struggle: too much medical intervention, too little care. She arrived at the emergency department on a Saturday night, clutching her abdomen in pain. At sixty-six, she had never been hospitalized and was in generally good health. But before she was even seen by a physician, she had to undergo an EKG, chest X-ray, CT scan with contrast, complete blood count, comprehensive metabolic panel, cardiac enzymes, D-dimer, urinalysis, and a series of other tests—a comprehensive diagnostic dragnet costing over $12,000. The final verdict? "Nonspecific abdominal pain."

When Linda came to see me the following week, looking bedraggled and still in pain, I had access to her entire emergency workup—a plethora of normal test results. What I didn't have—and what no one in the ER had asked her about—was her story. "What's happening in your life?" I asked her.

Linda explained that her mother, in the throes of Alzheimer's disease, had moved in with her three months prior. Linda had been managing her mother's care while working full-time and supporting her adult daughter who suffered from anxiety. Her sleep had been disrupted by worry over her mother's nighttime confusion and her daughter's lack of access to therapy. To compensate for her exhaustion, she was drinking more coffee, taking Advil by the fistful for tension headaches, and skipping lunch to get work done.

It didn't take a medical degree to figure out why her belly hurt: Linda was at the end of her rope. No CT scanner, however advanced, could visualize the physical effects of caregiver stress. No blood test could quantify sleep deprivation. No EKG could detect the heartache of constant worry. For Linda, the solution wasn't more tests; it was a combination of listening and offering support. It was educating her about how the stomach's sensitive lining can become irritated by the combination of stress, coffee, and Advil. We also reviewed some simple neck exercises and breathing techniques to help prevent tension headaches, to limit her reliance on Advil.

We discussed strategies to manage her mother's dementia care, and I connected her with a caregiver support group. What Linda needed most was a practical plan to reclaim a sense of agency over her health. Two weeks later, her belly pain had resolved. Her home responsibilities hadn't changed, but at least she felt empowered to care for herself first.

These two stories illustrate the central challenge of modern healthcare. Through no fault of doctors, our current medical system prioritizes transactions over relationships. It isn't designed to see you as a whole person or understand the relevance of your thoughts, feelings, and everyday behaviors to your health.

To anyone feeling disenfranchised from the US medical system, I feel your pain.

We all want to have access to high-quality healthcare and doctors who listen. We all want a sense of well-being. Despite remarkable technological advances—genetic sequencing, three-dimensional images of beating hearts, the ability to test for thousands of biomarkers—our healthcare system all too readily misses the human element. With so many medical messengers out there, it's hard to know who to trust. And when the average person doesn't feel well, they frequently don't know where to turn—a doctor who can see them in two weeks? The local Minute Clinic? Online experts or ChatGPT?

If you're lucky enough to have a primary care doctor who knows you, you might get a few minutes of their time—a hurried review of symptoms, a quick listen to your heart and lungs, a glance at your lab values, and a prescription on the way out. You might leave with blood pressure medication but no advice on various lifestyle changes to help bring your blood pressure down, and no insight into the root causes. You might get advice to "lose weight" or "eat more protein" without a plan that works for you.

But what does "wellness" even mean? What is "health," really? If you haven't stopped to consider what you are trying to achieve and how you are hoping to feel, how could a doctor or wellness guru possibly help you? These definitions matter, especially as we reckon with medical misinformation, chronic disease, and a broken healthcare system. Americans are sicker and heavier and more addicted—to sugar, alcohol, and screens—than ever before. We scroll through social media for wellness memes and quick hits of medical advice. We are irritable and sleepless and don't know what's wrong.

And yet, the solution isn't always more tests or prescriptions. Sometimes you don't need more testing; you just need someone to listen. Sometimes you don't need another prescription; you just need practical advice that fits your lifestyle. Yet through no fault of individual doctors, our healthcare system rarely creates space for these essential conversations. What's worse is that the conveyor-belt approach to medical care leaves patients feeling misunderstood and bewildered about whom to trust.

I understand this dilemma from both sides. As a first-year medical student at Harvard, I remember my first "patient-doctor" class vividly. Into our classroom walked a middle-aged man, an actor in a black tracksuit with pink leg warmers, ready to help us practice delivering difficult news. When my turn came to tell our mock patient that he had advanced prostate cancer, I felt both terrified and deeply moved. I took a deep breath and looked him straight in the eyes. My gaze softened, and so did his. More than anything else we had studied, establishing rapport and conveying life-changing information to vulnerable people felt meaningful in a way I hadn't anticipated. I left the class thinking: Being a doctor is going to require a lot more than "book" knowledge; it's about human connection first.

Yet during my training, both at Harvard and Johns Hopkins, I saw how humanism in medicine can evaporate in the face of what I call "medical maximalism." I recall performing CPR on a young woman who was dying of ovarian cancer—tubes and monitors everywhere, her family sobbing in the waiting room. When I later learned that neither she nor her family had been offered hospice care—the possibility of facing death with dignity at home rather than in an ICU—as an option, I felt a profound disillusionment. We were treating the cancer, not the human being.

For me, that moment crystallized a fundamental truth: Healthcare today excels at fighting diseases but too often fails to care for the people who have them. I get it. Doctors are trained to see a problem and fix it. Cancer cells? Chemotherapy. Infection? Antibiotics. Heart stopped? CPR. This approach has given us miraculous cures and saved countless lives. But it has also created a system that leaves little room for listening to the reasons our patients are alive in the first place.

Into this void has stepped the $4.4 trillion wellness industry. "Come hither!" it beckons. "I see you! I know your doctor has failed you!" And it's not wrong. The wellness industry, with its glossy marketing and the promise of youthful transformation, sells pseudoscience and lifestyle hacks that most mortals cannot sustain or afford. Yet despite the enormous profits flowing to pharmaceutical executives, insurance companies, and wellness influencers, Americans have never been sicker. These parallel systems profit from our continued suffering rather than addressing its root causes.

But there is hope. There is a middle path, one that integrates evidence-based medicine with a genuine understanding of who you are and what you need. This isn't about choosing sides in false battles between "natural" and "pharmaceutical" or between data and intuition; it's about reclaiming your role as the central decision maker in your own health story. After twenty-five years as a primary care doctor, I've witnessed patients navigate these systems successfully by developing what I call *health agency*—the ability to make informed decisions aligned with their values while effectively advocating for their needs. This requires a framework, not more rules or prescriptions.

I've developed a five-step process that will help you take charge of your health: redefine health on your terms, map your health ecosystem, understand your patient personality, ask for help effectively, and practice acceptance of what cannot be changed while focusing energy on what you can influence. The goal isn't to achieve perfection or abandon conventional medicine; it's to reclaim agency over your health. I'm not offering a quick fix or anything prescriptive; I'm offering a process to help you get what you need from our broken healthcare system and beckoning wellness industry and make smart decisions aligned with your priorities and values.

At its core, health should not be something that happens *to* you; it is something that happens inside you. Your health is yours to engage with actively, thoughtfully, and with intention. Whether you're managing a chronic condition, navigating a new diagnosis, or simply trying to feel better amid life's complexities, this book is your guide to answering the question all too rarely asked in modern healthcare: "Are you okay?"

1

How Did We Get Here?

"My mother had breast cancer—can I take hormone replacement therapy?"

"My orthopedist says I need surgery—should I trust him?"

"I can't get in to see my cardiologist for weeks—is this chest pain serious?"

These messages land in my inbox daily from newsletter subscribers and people in my community who don't have anyone else to ask—legitimate questions that could easily be answered by a primary care doctor with time. (Messages from my own patients are of course mine to answer!) Because so many Americans lack a primary care doctor or medical "home," they don't know where to turn for basic questions or routine care. Instead, they end up in emergency rooms for problems that could be resolved by an accessible primary care physician, or they reach out to doctors like me through whatever channels they can find. When I worked in the Johns Hopkins emergency room, my colleagues and I weren't just providing emergency care; we were effectively serving as primary care providers for East Baltimore—treating diabetics who couldn't afford insulin, asthmatics who'd never developed management plans, and elderly patients with urinary tract infections who lacked access to basic preventive care. But increasingly today, even in well-resourced areas, more and more people lack access to basic health guidance.

How did we reach this point? America faces a paradoxical health crisis: unprecedented access to medical information alongside declining health outcomes. Despite technological advances and trillion-dollar industries focused on health, US life expectancy lags significantly behind that of other wealthy nations. Six in ten Americans have at least one chronic disease,[1] over 40 percent have obesity,[2] and mental health conditions affect one in five adults in any given year.[3] Meanwhile, as of 2023, more than 100 million Americans—nearly one-third of the population—face barriers to accessing primary care due to provider shortages in their communities.[4]

How did caring for our health become a healthcare system that seems to have fundamentally lost its way?

How Electronic Health Records Broke Healthcare

Primary care physicians face impossible demands; they must see twenty to twenty-five patients daily in fifteen-minute slots while extensively documenting each condition and visit for insurance requirements. This assembly-line approach leaves little room for understanding patients' stories or addressing the root causes of problems. One study found that on average, doctors interrupt patients within eleven seconds after a patient starts to speak.

Electronic health records (EHRs) were meant to improve efficiency and patient outcomes but have instead turned relationships into transac-

---

1 Timothy Jay Carney et al., "Advancing Chronic Disease Practice Through the CDC Data Modernization Initiative," *Preventing Chronic Disease* 20 (November 20, 2023), https://www.cdc.gov/pcd/issues/2023/23_0120.htm.

2 Gabriel A. Benavidez et al., "Chronic Disease Prevalence in the US: Sociodemographic and Geographic Variations by Zip Code Tabulation Area," *Preventing Chronic Disease* 21 (February 29, 2024), https://www.cdc.gov/pcd/issues/2024/23_0267.htm.

3 "Mental Illness," National Institute of Mental Health, updated September 2024, https://www.nimh.nih.gov/health/statistics/mental-illness.

4 "Closing the Primary Care Gap: How Community Health Centers Can Address the Nation's Primary Care Crisis," National Association of Community Health Centers, updated February 7, 2023, https://www.nachc.org/resource/closing-the-primary-care-gap-how-community-health-centers-can-address-the-nations-primary-care-crisis/.

tions. Physicians now spend two hours on documentation for every hour they spend with patients; doctors' eyes are fixed on screens instead of on faces. When all the administrative tasks are included, only 27 percent of a doctor's time is spent with patients. Emergency room doctors, who make an average of four thousand EHR system clicks per shift, report the highest levels of burnout. Primary care physicians spend an estimated one to two hours every night after work finishing up their data entry on EHRs. By forcing clinicians to focus on screens rather than patients, this technology jeopardizes the already-fragile patient-doctor relationship, reducing human experiences to data points and billing codes.

Most aggravating for patients and providers alike is that EHRs lack real-time updating across healthcare systems. If you get a tetanus booster at an urgent care clinic while on vacation, that vital information often never makes it into your primary doctor's records. Lab results from one hospital don't automatically appear in another hospital's system. Several doctors treating the same patient may be working from entirely different—and sometimes conflicting—EHR data. Even worse, most EHRs lack an essential component: a shared care plan. Without this, there's no centralized strategy for managing a patient's various medical problems, no clear implementation steps, and no accessible document that patients can share with new providers. An ER doctor treating your chest pain can't access your cardiac history, your current medications, or the treatment goals established by your cardiologist.

In addition, EHRs don't elicit important elements of patients' life experiences that directly affect their risks for disease and treatment outcomes. Until the EHR is reinvented to include more relevant details about the patient's social-emotional health, goals, life circumstances, and preferences, these systems remain incomplete repositories of faceless data rather than true representations of the person. And too few doctors have enough training and/or time to fill in the blanks. Consider my patient Susan, a forty-two-year-old professional with persistent migraines. After seeing three specialists and undergoing numerous scans, she was prescribed medications during an urgent care visit and later by a neurologist, but she had no clear record of what each doctor had given her, and neither physician knew about the other's prescriptions. The medications turned out to interact negatively, worsening her symptoms.

Meanwhile, Susan's patient portal pinged with a notification: Her brain MRI results were available on the hospital EHR. What she saw terrified her: "nonspecific white matter changes" with no explanation, no context, and no way to reach her neurologist for clarification. So she did what millions of other people do every day: She turned to Google. Within minutes, she'd convinced herself that she had multiple sclerosis. Her headaches intensified as anxiety compounded her physical symptoms.

When we finally met in my office, she was visibly upset—jaw tense, eyes wide with fear. I did a full neurologic exam and sat with her to review her MRI images together. I explained that her brain was normal and that the "nonspecific changes" she'd read about were simply reflections of her long history of migraines—a common benign finding that her neurologist should have told her about.

But here's what no test or EHR could reveal: Susan's manager at work had been harassing her for months. Her migraines had started flaring up within weeks of that toxic situation. The combination of tight neck and jaw muscles due to stress, plus long days sitting anxiously at her desk, had triggered a cascade of neurological symptoms. No imaging study could detect the connection between her emotional distress and her physical pain, yet addressing the toxic work situation proved to be more effective than any medication.

Susan's experience reveals how our fragmented and impersonal system fails patients in several ways: She received her test results without context, leaving her to connect the dots with internet searches and worst-case scenarios. Her doctors focused on ruling out serious pathology while missing the obvious trigger for her symptoms. Most critically, she had no central figure—no primary care partner—to help her make sense of conflicting information, coordinate her care, and develop a comprehensive plan that would address both her medical needs and her life circumstances.

This is what happens when we reduce patients to data points while ignoring the human experiences that drive illness: We don't just provide inadequate care, we disempower them.

For doctors like me, the choices have become stark: Stay in a system that rewards volume over relationships and prescriptions over prevention, find a way to practice medicine differently, or leave the profession entirely. Increasingly, many are choosing the last two options. The exodus is real and accelerating. A 2024 survey by the Medical Group Management Association (MGMA)[5] found that 27 percent of physician groups reported that a doctor left or retired early in 2024 due to burnout. Every day, talented physicians abandon clinical practice to become administrators, consultants, or anything else that allows them to alleviate the moral injury of providing suboptimal care due to systemic constraints.

The US faces a looming physician shortage, projected to be up to 124,000 by 2034.[6] Doctors who remain often do so by creating alternative practice models—concierge medicine, direct primary care, cash-only practices—that allow them to spend time with patients. But these solutions, while better for the doctors and patients who can access them, inadvertently worsen the crisis by removing experienced physicians from the broader system, leaving even fewer doctors available for everyone else.

The human cost is staggering. Physicians report depression rates twice that of the general population. Suicide rates among doctors exceed those of any other profession. We're losing not just individual careers but institutional knowledge and expertise that takes decades to develop. When the healers are sicker than the patients they're supposed to treat, the system isn't just broken, it's actively harmful to everyone it touches. This isn't sustainable.

---

5 Chris Harrop, "Physician Burnout Still a Major Factor Even as Unexpected Turnover Eases," Medical Group Management Association, September 4, 2024, https://www.mgma.com/mgma-stat/physician-burnout-still-major-factor-even-as-unexpected-turnover-eases.

6 "AAMC Report Reinforces Mounting Physician Shortage," Association of American Medical Colleges, updated June 11, 2021, https://www.aamc.org/news/press-releases/aamc-report-reinforces-mounting-physician-shortage.

What Healthcare Could Look Like (If We Actually Fixed It)

But what if we could flip this equation? What if technology, instead of creating barriers between doctors and patients, could eliminate them? What if artificial intelligence could handle the administrative burden that currently consumes physicians' time and attention, freeing them to do what they trained for: understand, diagnose, and heal?

Imagine walking into a primary care office where your doctor spends the entire appointment looking at you, not at a screen. Behind the scenes, AI has already synthesized your latest lab results, updated your medications across all systems, flagged potential drug interactions, and prepared a detailed report of all outside records and specialists' recommendations. Your tetanus shot from that urgent care visit last month? It was automatically integrated into your record. The chest pain you mentioned to the cardiologist? Your primary care doctor already knows about it. Then together you and your doctor create a personalized treatment plan that no AI agent could arrive at.

This isn't science fiction; it's an achievable vision that puts human connection back at the center of healthcare while leveraging technology to solve the problems that plague the system.

In this reimagined primary care model, every patient would have access to a medical home that serves as a hub for problem-solving, not gatekeeping. Your primary care doctor wouldn't just be someone who refers you elsewhere when problems arise, they would be equipped with intelligent systems to help them coordinate your care, track your progress toward health goals, and anticipate issues before they become crises.

Most important, you would have a shared care plan—not just a list of diagnoses buried in an EHR but a living document that outlines your health goals, strategies for achieving them, and built-in checkpoints along the way. This plan would be visible to you, your doctor, and any specialists or emergency physicians who treat you. It would evolve as your health changes, always reflecting your current priorities and circumstances. If you end up in an emergency room at 2:00 a.m., the doctor treating you would instantly understand not just your medical history but your health goals and preferences for care.

This transformation would fundamentally change what it means to be a patient. Instead of being a passive recipient of fragmented care, you would be an active partner in a coherent health strategy. Instead of having to repeat your medical history to every new provider, you would have a comprehensive record that would travel with you. Instead of wondering whether your doctors are communicating with one another, you would see the coordination happening in real time.

For physicians, this model would restore the joy of practicing medicine. Instead of spending their evenings typing notes and clicking boxes, doctors could focus on the intellectual challenges and human connections that drew them to medicine in the first place. The moral injury of providing suboptimal care due to time constraints would diminish as technology handles routine tasks and doctors have adequate time with each patient.

This isn't just about making healthcare more pleasant, it's about making it more effective. When primary care physicians have the tools and time to get to know their patients, they catch problems earlier, prevent more serious illnesses, and help people maintain health rather than just treating disease. The result is better outcomes, lower costs, and a healthcare system that serves human flourishing.

The technology to create this reality already exists. What we need now is the will to demand it—by patients who refuse to accept the current broken system, by doctors who remember why they became physicians, and by leaders who understand that healthcare transformation isn't just possible, it's essential.

This is why your role as an active, informed healthcare advocate matters more than ever. By understanding what healthcare could be and demanding better from the system, you will become part of the movement toward a future in which primary care works the way it should: with human connection at the center and technology as the invisible assistant that makes everything else possible.

But there is another reason why medicine must experience this transformation. Medical care is being replaced by a new movement that promises health in the guise of "wellness" but too often delivers neither.

How Wellness Culture Profits from Your Suffering

As patients increasingly feel abandoned by conventional medicine, the wellness industry has seized the advantage, branding itself as medicine's enlightened alternative. Unlike healthcare's sterile waiting rooms and rushed appointments, wellness is sleek, accessible, and designed to make you feel seen and understood. It speaks to our deepest desires: Vitality! Longevity! Control!

But let's be clear about what we're dealing with: This is a $6.3 trillion global industry—four times larger than the pharmaceutical industry—that profits handsomely from selling you hope without accountability. In the United States alone, Americans spend $480 billion annually on wellness products and services, a number that is growing by 5 to 10 percent each year even during times of economic uncertainty. We spend nearly 60 percent as much on wellness products as we do on all traditional healthcare combined.[7] We're talking about an industry larger than IT, sports, tourism, and the green economy combined. These numbers are the result of sophisticated marketing that deliberately targets our deepest fears and insecurities.

The wellness industry's messaging is seductive: You can control your destiny and improve your health through willpower and the right products. The problem is that much of what wellness culture sells is un-

7 Shaun Callaghan et al., "Still Feeling Good: The US Wellness Market Continues to Boom," McKinsey & Company, updated September 19, 2022, https://www.mckinsey.com/industries/consumer-packaged-goods/our-insights/still-feeling-good-the-us-wellness-market-continues-to-boom#/.

proven; much of its advice isn't evidence based. The irony is that wellness is as prescriptive as its medical counterparts—just with better marketing and far more dangerous implications. Its core message is that health is achievable through discipline and consumption: Track your sleep, optimize your gut microbiome, detoxify your system, and take the right supplements. The underlying assumption? Perfect health is possible if you only try hard enough.

Here's the fundamental lie that's making billionaires out of wellness gurus: You cannot biohack your way to immortality. You cannot optimize your way out of genetics, bad luck, or the reality that our bodies break down despite our best efforts. The wellness industry wants you to believe that if you just eat enough superfoods, take enough supplements, and follow its strict protocols, you will be healthy. This isn't just false; it's harmful, and it's designed to keep you buying.

This narrative is sexy because it contains partial truths. Nutrition does matter. Movement is beneficial. Sleep is essential. Mindfulness has value. But wellness culture weaponizes these truths, suggesting that they're sufficient when they're merely foundational. You can eat organic kale for decades and still develop colon cancer. You can meditate daily and still need blood pressure medication. You can optimize your gut microbiome and still face a devastating diagnosis that has nothing to do with your wellness routine. More problematically, wellness has become a status symbol that is accessible primarily to those with time, money, and privilege. It profits from people's anxieties. It sells solutions to nonproblems. It steers people away from consulting medical doctors and getting the care they genuinely need.

The supplement industry alone, operating with minimal oversight, generates over $50 billion yearly selling products that may contain undisclosed pharmaceutical ingredients, heavy metals, or compounds not listed on labels. Here's what that money is buying: Between 2007 and 2016, the Food and Drug Administration (FDA) found nearly a thousand products masquerading as dietary supplements that contained active pharmaceutical compounds from prescription drugs.[8] About one-third of sports performance supplements contained steroids, hormone modulators, and/or stimulants not listed on their labels. These undisclosed ingredients can cause liver damage, heart problems, and dangerous drug interactions—all while consumers believe that they're taking something "natural" and safe.

The human cost is real and measurable. Nearly twenty-three thousand people visit emergency rooms annually because of adverse reactions to dietary supplements. In a national survey, one in eight adults reported that they or an immediate family member had experienced extreme side effects—increased heart rate, high blood pressure, kidney problems, or liver damage—as a result of taking dietary supplements. Yet 40 percent of patients don't even tell their doctors what supplements they're taking.

What wellness culture calls personal empowerment is a fantasy that can literally kill you.

I've seen the real-world consequences of this messaging on a patient who delayed breast cancer treatment to try alkaline water and coffee enemas. A diabetic who stopped taking insulin because a wellness guru convinced her she could reverse her condition through intermittent fasting alone. A man with heart disease who refused statins because he'd been told that pharmaceuticals were "toxic" but willingly took unregulated supplements that interacted dangerously with his other medications.

Health technology exemplifies this double-edged sword. A patient once described her fitness tracker as "a bad boyfriend," constantly demanding more while making her feel increasingly inadequate. Another patient with an expensive sleep tracker developed insomnia from obsessing over her sleep scores, exactly the opposite of the device's intended purpose. These aren't isolated cases; they're predictable outcomes of an industry that profits from anxiety and inadequacy.

---

8 Jenna Tucker et al., "Unapproved Pharmaceutical Ingredients Included in Dietary Supplements Associated with US Food and Drug Administration Warnings," *JAMA Netw Open* 1 (6): e183337 (October 12, 2018), https://pmc.ncbi.nlm.nih.gov/articles/PMC6324457/.

The most insidious aspect of wellness culture is how it privatizes health outcomes, suggesting that illness is fundamentally a personal failure. Can't lose weight? You're not disciplined enough. Developed diabetes? You didn't optimize your diet sufficiently. Need medication? You're taking the easy way out instead of doing the hard work of healing naturally. This framework doesn't just ignore the reality of how disease works; it actively harms people by adding shame to suffering.

Let me be clear: There's nothing wrong with wanting to feel good, eat well, move your body, or understand how your choices affect your health, but the wellness industry doesn't want you healthy; it wants you hopeful, anxious, and purchasing. Because the moment you achieve the health you're seeking, you stop being profitable to them.

It's Time to Take Control of Your Health

Neither system—conventional medicine or wellness culture—meets our needs. The medical system struggles to see the person behind the data. The wellness industry sells products and false hope without accountability. I regularly see patients caught between these two worlds. Take Laura, a woman in her mid-fifties with obesity who had tried every diet without success. Every doctor had taken one look at her weight and repeated the same refrain: "Eat less, move more," without listening to her story. She left each appointment feeling judged and lost. So she had done what people do: She combed the internet. After trying several diets and supplements promising metabolic miracles, she gave up. When I saw her for the first time, I needed to understand her as a person first. After we established rapport, she revealed in a follow-up visit that she'd been a victim of sexual assault in her twenties. To cope with the secrecy and pain, she had started using food for comfort. Her weight problem was never going to be solved by a stern lecture or another strict diet; she needed help to break a vicious cycle of shame and binge eating.

Or consider James, a forty-eight-year-old with high blood pressure who refused medication, determined to reduce his blood pressure with mindfulness and herbal supplements instead. The wellness industry and influencers such as Joe Rogan had convinced him that Big Pharma "owned" medical doctors and that "real men" eschewed prescription medication. One morning after consuming a caffeine-rich protein drink, he lost his ability to speak. In the ER, his blood pressure was 190/110 mmHg, and his brain MRI showed he had suffered a minor stroke. By the time we met, James realized he'd been sold a lie by the online wellness "manosphere." What he'd thought was empowerment was dangerous ideology that nearly killed him. He didn't need more products; he needed blood pressure medication, a trusted guide, and a road map.

Each patient had been failed by both medicine and wellness. They needed a middle path, a nuanced plan that sees medications not as moral failures but as tools to create space for sustainable behavior changes; a plan that acknowledges that lifestyle directly impacts health outcomes, but so do genetics, environmental factors, past experiences, and plain old bad luck. This isn't about rejecting all wellness practices or dismissing the value of lifestyle changes; it's about rejecting the false promises that exercise or diet or mindfulness alone can prevent disease or that you can optimize your way out of medical problems. It's about acknowledging both the power and the limitations of personal agency in health. Instead of falling victim to these deeply flawed and equally prescriptive industries, I'm advocating for a framework that combines the best of evidence-based medicine with the science-backed lifestyle wisdom that wellness culture emphasizes. This integrated approach centers *you*—not as a collection of symptoms or lab values, not as a consumer of wellness products, but as a whole person making informed decisions about your health within the context of your real life, your real body, and the real world. Let's face it: Genetics and green smoothies matter, but neither one alone determines your fate.

You deserve better than a healthcare system that reduces you to data points, and you deserve better than a wellness industry that sells you the illusion of control. If you're ready to reclaim agency over your health, you are in the right place. If you're ready to navigate our broken healthcare system with more confidence, keep reading.

2

Becoming the CEO of Your Own Health

Imagine standing at a crossroads. On one path, health is something done *to* you—a series of prescriptions, test results, and recommendations you passively receive. On the other, health is something you actively shape, a dynamic process that you lead based on your unique needs, values, and circumstances. This chapter is about choosing the second path.

When it comes to health, most of us find ourselves caught in a cycle of good intentions and missed opportunities. We strive to exercise, eat well, and manage stress, yet when our life intensifies—when work deadlines loom, our children get sick, or our aging parents need help—we default to survival mode. The sugar cravings return. The wine bottle beckons us to relax. Screen time replaces sleep time. And tomorrow, we promise ourselves, we'll do better.

This cycle isn't due to a failure of willpower; it's the inevitable result of approaching health without a personalized framework, one that accounts for who you truly are, what your life is really like, and what you genuinely need. When health becomes a collection of disconnected "shoulds" rather than an integrated expression of your values and the realities of your own life, it remains forever fragile, collapsing under life's predictable and unpredictable pressures.

I know this cycle intimately, both as a doctor and as a patient. In college, I struggled with anxiety, depression, and disordered eating. To most observers, I looked like a typical slender coed, but beneath the mirage of fitness and "health" was a scared and miserable young woman. My bodily systems were constantly dysregulated. My heart raced, my head pounded. I had digestive issues, cold sweats, and hair loss.

Doctors tested me for everything from parasites to brain tumors. Every test came back normal. Rather than feeling reassured, I felt more anxious. What were they missing? When I sought help from my university psychologist, she told me that I was doing fine academically, had a loving family and boyfriend, and should just continue my running routine to relieve stress. So I did, losing weight and feeling even sicker.

It wasn't until medical school, after a family friend died and I couldn't stop crying for two weeks, that I finally found a therapist who helped me see the connections among my anxiety, restrictive eating, and physical symptoms. The most profound things she gave me were permission to be human and a prescription for self-compassion.

That experience taught me something that medical textbooks couldn't: that health is not a collection of normal test results or physical metrics; it is the intersection of physical, emotional, and spiritual well-being—a complex ecosystem in which every part communicates with every other part. It is, fundamentally, about relationships: the relationship between body and mind, between conscious and unconscious thought, between our past experiences and present choices, between ourselves and those who care for us.

Listening to my patients and to myself is how and why I've developed this five-step process to help you reclaim agency over your health. This frame provides some "prework" you might do before visiting your primary care doctor. It is designed to help you squeeze the most out of the medical system and to better advocate for yourself within it. I hope it opens your mind to what is possible for you (and for the future of healthcare in this country!). As you go through the five steps, I suggest grabbing a pen and paper to jot down notes, doodle, and dream big.

Let's get started.

Step 1: Redefine Health on Your Own Terms

Let's start with a fundamental question: What does "health" mean to you?

When I ask my patients this question, it often stops them in their tracks. My younger patients will reply with something such as "I eat pretty clean, is that what you mean?" My elderly patients say things such as "Being with my family is all that matters" or "I'm just glad to be alive." But the most common reply? "Doctor, you have my lab results. How do I look?"

It's clear to me that people have been socialized to measure their health by someone else's standards. We are conditioned to define health as something outside ourselves, sometimes *external* and measurable only through lab tests and metrics. A normal mammogram. An optimal cholesterol score. A clean CT scan. Yes, I'm a doctor and test results matter, but it's time to understand that metrics cannot capture what health really is.

It may take you a minute to figure out what I'm asking. Take your time, because everything else flows from here. Remember this: Defining health for yourself doesn't require spreadsheets or glamorous plans; it starts by tuning in to what matters most to you today. This first step is about defining your North Star: your core values, your vision for your future, the reasons you get out of bed in the morning. Maybe it involves regaining your strength after surgery or illness. Maybe it involves starting an exercise program or challenging your social anxiety. Maybe it involves waking up in the morning and not dreading the day ahead.

Whether you know it or not, your priorities already inform your health in important ways, from the everyday risks you undertake to the major medical trade-offs you make. You may understand that alcohol consumption increases the risk of developing breast cancer but enjoy a few drinks anyway. You may choose pain medications over knee surgery because missing your daily hikes during post-op recovery isn't worth the cost to your emotional health right now. I'm asking you to name your priorities and core values. Otherwise the healthcare system will assume what they are or, worse, name them for you. Without reckoning with what you want and what makes you *you*, you're at the mercy of someone else's health map. You risk falling victim to someone else's definition of health.

This is exactly what happened to Jenna, a forty-two-year-old marketing executive. By conventional standards, she was the picture of "health": running half-marathons, tracking her sleep with a smartwatch, diligently following her wellness coach's supplement regimen. Yet she came to me feeling exhausted, with persistent migraines and escalating anxiety. She woke up most mornings feeling as though she was sprinting toward an invisible finish line. "I've tried everything," she told me, detailing her visits to numerous doctors, nutritionists, and a functional medicine specialist. Her labs were perfect. Her vital signs and physical exam were normal. Yet she felt terrible.

"What does being healthy mean to you?" I asked her.

"I guess I just want to enjoy the moment every now and then," she replied. Until that moment, she had never considered *contentedness* as an essential element of health or known that subconsciously she had outsourced her definition of health to someone else. Adherence to rigid standards and arbitrary goals was exhausting her. Not questioning the trade-offs and not asking herself what mattered to her was the root cause of her headaches and anxiety symptoms. What she needed most was a broader understanding of health.

This isn't just my opinion; it's supported by the way health experts think about wellness more broadly. The World Health Organization (WHO) defines "health" as "a state of complete physical, mental, and social well-being and not merely the absence of disease or infirmity." The same concept applies to your own health. *Your* definition should stem from your core beliefs and values. Reasonable people can disagree on what risks are worth taking and what trade-offs are worth making. Medicine's job isn't to define health for someone else; it's to help people make decisions using each person's North Star as the guide.

A note on language: Throughout this book, when I refer to "health"—whether it is physical health, mental health, or cognitive health—I mean a state of well-being as *you* define it. I intentionally avoided saying "good health" or "bad health" because health itself is a goal you're working toward based on your own values and circumstances. When I say "redefine health on your terms" or "improve your mental health," the "good" is implicit—it's whatever version of well-being aligns with your North Star. However, qualifying health with the word "good" suggests there's a universal standard we should all chase, or that health has a specific definition, which are the very assumptions that I'm asking you to question. Far from being a fixed data point, health is a dynamic state that will shift with your priorities, circumstances, and season of life. So, when you read "health" in these pages, understand it to mean: *well-being as you define it, given your unique informatics, values, and the trade-offs you're willing to make.*

For Darcy, defining health on her own terms became particularly crucial at the end of her life. A fifty-eight-year-old teacher with advanced cancer, she was facing hard decisions: Should she undergo another round of aggressive chemotherapy with serious side effects or prioritize comfort care? There was no right answer; there was only the answer that made sense for her. Informed about the trade-offs inherent in her decision and based on our mutual understanding of what gave her life meaning, she chose to forgo more chemotherapy and opted for home hospice care. A few weeks later, she died peacefully in her own bed, surrounded by loved ones. It was her decision, aligned with her values, and therefore it was the right one for her.

There are no solutions in health, only trade-offs that reflect your priorities. So when a patient asks me, "*Can* I do X?" or "*Should* I do Y?" my answer isn't a hard yes or no. Instead, I try to reframe their questions to "What are the inherent risks and benefits of doing X?" or "What are the trade-offs of not doing Y?" My patients' health is not about me, my values, or my tolerance for risk—it's about theirs. The best clinical decisions occur when doctors apply medical data and center the patient's preferences, instead of assuming what the patient wants or basing their decisions on their own personal preferences.

Redefine Health on Your Own Terms

Throughout this book, and as you embark on the process of self-empowerment, I will invite you to various "thought exercises." I suggest grabbing a pen and paper or opening a blank page on your laptop. Over the course of these pages, you develop the framework to better understand and evaluate your health. By the end, you will have a smarter, more accurate rendering of your health to bring to every medical encounter.

Let's start with definitions. To redefine health on your own terms, consider these fundamental questions about your health. (This isn't a test; there are no right answers!) Are you ready?

- Imagine yourself ten years from now. What does a "healthy" version of you look like? What is that person doing, feeling, and prioritizing?
- What are five adjectives that taken together describe your personal definition of "good health"? (e.g., "fit," "pain-free," "less depressed," "active," "socially engaged," "rested," "less stressed," "unmedicated," "natural," "cancer-free," "accepting of my mortality")
- Does your definition of health feel authentic and true to you? Or is your definition tied to someone else's definition of your health? If so, whose?
- Is your definition of health realistic and attainable, or purely aspirational?
- How do the current realities of your life (health, finances, social-emotional stress, work/parenting/caregiving responsibilities) inform your definition of health?
- How do the realities of your life help or hinder your ability to be "healthy" according to your definition?
- What are the biggest trade-offs you're currently making to meet your health goals (e.g. sleeping less to get to the gym before work or taking a prescription medication that has unpleasant side effects)? How do you decide what is "worth it"?
- Have you ever sacrificed your well-being pursuing someone else's health goal—losing weight for a doctor or partner, adopting a fitness routine to fit in with your social group, or fixing a health problem you didn't actually have? What did you learn about yourself?

- How do you measure success in your health "journey"? What would it feel like—physically and emotionally—to feel healthier tomorrow than you do today?

Step 1 is now underway. Defining health on your own terms sets the stage for understanding the complexities of your health. (Hint: It's about more than your cholesterol levels and weight.)

Step 2: Map Your Health Ecosystem

Now that you've drilled down into what "health" means for you, the next step is to understand the core elements of your health. This is not about isolated body parts or pieces of data; it's about the relationships among the various parts of your health: body and mind, nutrition and movement, cognition and emotional health. It means that your blood pressure is affected by your job stress and sleeplessness as much as it is by your blood pressure pills. It means that working on your relationship with food may help you lose weight more than any strict diet will. It requires recognizing the relevance of your childhood experiences to your health habits as an adult. It involves recognizing the connections among your medical data, your genetics, your environment, and how you feel. Understanding these relationships can help you build a strategic plan to improve your health. By teaching you this new framework, I hope to hand you the power to shape your well-being.

Your health ecosystem consists of four interdependent quadrants:

INFORMATICS: Your medical data *and* your biographic data (i.e., your life story). This includes the traditional measurements doctors collect—lab tests, vital signs, imaging results—alongside the facts of your life and all of your experiences. It's not only your gender and genetic predispositions but also your childhood experiences, significant relationships, and cultural context. It's both the "city's" official records and its unwritten history.

INPUTS: Everything you consume, from food and water to medications, supplements, alcohol, and anything else that enters your body. These are the resources flowing through your "city," determining your energy levels, cellular function, and biochemical balance. Each input carries meaning and consequences, informing not just your physical state but your emotional landscape as well.

INFRASTRUCTURE: Your physical container; your skeleton and your complex body mechanics. This is the framework that carries you through life—your bones, muscles, tendons, and fascia. Like a city's infrastructure, your body requires ongoing maintenance and occasional repairs. Understanding your body's particular architecture—your asymmetries, past injuries, and movement patterns—is crucial for maintaining mobility and preventing breakdown.

INSIGHT: Your inner landscape. This is where your mental and emotional health reside in your fears, beliefs, unconscious patterns, and the stories you tell yourself. It's the collective consciousness of your internal "city," informing how you respond to stress, process emotions, and relate to yourself and others. This quadrant requires honesty, courage, and curiosity about what you don't yet know about yourself.

What makes this approach transformative isn't just the individual quadrants themselves; it's the way each part influences and is influenced by every other part. Health improves not by optimizing isolated quadrants but through understanding the relationships between them. This ecosystem approach doesn't just lead to better outcomes, it empowers patients by helping them understand that they have numerous pathways toward meeting their health goals.

My patient Tom illustrates this interconnectedness perfectly. A sixty-two-year-old college professor, he came to me because his diabetes was spiraling out of control. His hemoglobin A1C diabetes marker was elevated at 8.5% despite years of stable management (INFORMATICS). It would have been easy for me simply to ratchet up his diabetes medication and send him on his way. But when I asked him about what had changed in his life, he admitted that he'd been avoiding social activities due to chronic back pain from an old injury that he'd been ignoring (INFRASTRUCTURE).

The untreated back pain had gradually isolated him from his colleagues and friends. He had stopped attending faculty gatherings, had quit taking his evening walks, and avoided standing for long periods while teaching. The social isolation and lack of exercise had triggered depression he didn't recognize until I asked him about his spirits (INSIGHT). Without his routines, he had become somewhat apathetic about his health, ordering takeout instead of cooking and sometimes skipping his diabetes medications (INPUTS). What seemed like a diabetes problem was actually an untreated musculoskeletal problem at its core.

"I don't think you need more diabetes medication to fix your A1C," I told him. "We need to address the root cause."

After a few weeks in physical therapy and with new walking shoes, Tom's back pain improved. As a result, his social engagement and mood gradually improved. He regained the motivation to maintain healthy habits. Within three months, his blood sugar level was back to normal with a hemoglobin A1C of 6.2%. Addressing his infrastructure problem had improved his diabetes control and restored his entire health ecosystem. Most important, he had developed a newfound sense of agency over his health.

This is the fundamental insight of the health ecosystem approach: Seemingly unrelated problems are often deeply connected, and addressing the root issue in one quadrant can create positive changes throughout your entire health landscape. We will spend the bulk of this book sketching out your health ecosystem and connecting the dots between the various elements. Keep your pen and paper handy!

Step 3: Understand Your Patient Personality

With your health redefined (step 1) and your ecosystem mapped (step 2), the next step to reclaiming your health is owning your unique approach to healthcare situations. This is what I call your "patient personality"—the set of biases, beliefs, fears, and knowledge you bring to every medical encounter, whether you are consulting a doctor or researching symptoms online.

Your patient personality informs how you process health information, respond to medical advice, and make healthcare decisions. It can either facilitate or obstruct your path to better health. I have a patient personality, too, and it can easily interfere with my health! (Ask me about how I ate a bagel ten minutes before my emergency appendectomy, causing my surgery to be postponed and my appendix to be gangrenous by the time it was taken out.)

The concept of having a patient personality isn't a medical diagnosis but a framework I've developed from two decades of observing how people interact with healthcare. I've witnessed even the best-informed patients get in their own way and seen vulnerable individuals bravely confront their biases to get the help they need.

In chapter 15 I will lay out some common patient personalities I've identified, including the **Optimizer**, who believes that perfect health is achievable through self-discipline and lifestyle optimization, often overlooking genetic factors or conditions that require medical intervention beyond lifestyle changes; the **Pleaser**, who defers to medical authorities and rarely questions recommendations, sometimes at the expense of their health; the **Internet Warrior**, who researches extensively, whose knowledge can be valuable but can also create anxiety; and the **Outsourcer**, an efficiency-minded patient who readily delegates medical decisions to experts, seeking quick solutions rather than understanding the "whys" or tolerating gray areas.

The key isn't to label or judge yourself but rather to understand how you engage with healthcare providers and how they might see you. Once you notice the patterns that influence your healthcare experiences, you can become a better advocate for yourself. Understanding your patient personality opens the next step on the path to improved agency: asking for help.

Step 4: Ask for Help

To be healthy is to seek support and guidance, yet asking for help remains challenging for many of us. The right help is not always available or accessible, not to mention that asking for help requires recognizing that you need it.

The healthcare landscape makes this particularly difficult. Whom should you trust? How should you navigate the maze of specialists, alternative practitioners, health coaches, and online experts? How can you separate evidence-based guidance from marketing hype? Most people don't have a doctor who can quarterback their care. So until every American has access to a good primary care doctor—a medical home in which doctors serve as their patients' chief medical advocates while providing medical care, preventive counseling, and care coordination among members of their team—getting the right help begins by identifying the elements of your health ecosystem that need support. Each area may require specific help: medical, psychological, social-emotional, nutritional, physical.

If you're having trouble making sense of your risk for heart disease, you may need a new primary care doctor. If Advil and rest aren't doing the trick for your bum knee, it's probably time to see a physical therapist. If you're struggling to lose weight, you might benefit from seeing a registered dietitian who can help you with emotional eating. If you're feeling anxious, you may need an exercise program or a good psychotherapist.

No one achieves health in isolation. Learning to ask for help strategically (and accept it gracefully) is essential to your health.

Step 5: Practice Acceptance

Acceptance is arguably the hardest part of being human. It involves the lifelong process of letting go of what we cannot control, including genetic predispositions, aging, past traumas, certain chronic conditions, and circumstances beyond our influence. This isn't resignation or giving up; it's the clear-eyed recognition of reality that allows us to focus our limited resources, time, energy, and money where they can make a difference. Paradoxically, true agency emerges from acceptance. When we stop fighting unwinnable battles, we discover where meaningful change is possible.

Consider the wisdom of the Serenity Prayer, which asks for "the serenity to accept the things I cannot change, courage to change the things I can, and wisdom to know the difference." This simple prayer captures the essence of health as a dynamic balance between acceptance and action. Acceptance is an ongoing practice requiring patience, self-compassion, and often guidance from others who have walked similar paths. This ongoing practice may involve grieving losses, distinguishing between what can and cannot be modified, and focusing attention where change is in fact possible.

Integrating the Five Steps

These five steps form an integrated framework for becoming the CEO of your own health. You'll cycle through these steps as your circumstances change, continuously refining how you understand and approach your health. In the next twelve chapters, we'll explore each quadrant of your health ecosystem. You'll learn to identify patterns, understand connections, and make decisions aligned with your values and circumstances.

You'll learn practical ways to apply this framework to your real life. Here's how the four quadrants and five steps work together:

Step 1—Redefine Health on Your Own Terms—sets your personal health vision and values.

Step 2—Map Your Health Ecosystem—is accomplished by understanding all four quadrants: INFORMATICS, INPUTS, INFRASTRUCTURE, and INSIGHT.

Step 3—Recognize Your Patient Personality—helps you navigate healthcare relationships across all quadrants.

Step 4—Ask for Help—helps you understand which quadrant (or quadrants) needs support and how to find it.

Step 5—Practice Acceptance—applies to limitations that you discover in each quadrant.

This framework works whether you have excellent access to healthcare or must navigate a fragmented system alone. I realize that many readers may not have a primary care provider to partner with and activate on the frame we're about to create.

If you're among those without a trusted medical guide, all is not lost; this framework just becomes more essential. Think of it as your personal health GPS. Just as a GPS can guide you to your destination whether you're driving a luxury car or taking public transportation, these five steps can guide your health decisions whether you have a concierge physician or rely on a community health center. The destination—better health aligned with your values—remains the same. The journey may look different depending on your resources, but the principles that guide smart health decisions remain constant.

Your health ecosystem doesn't pause because you lack a regular doctor. Your body doesn't stop being complex because you have limited access to healthcare. In fact, understanding how your INFORMATICS, INPUTS, INFRASTRUCTURE, and INSIGHT quadrants interconnect becomes even more crucial when you're piecing together care from various sources. This knowledge will transform you from a passive recipient of fragmented care into an active coordinator of your own well-being.

Are you ready to start mapping your health?

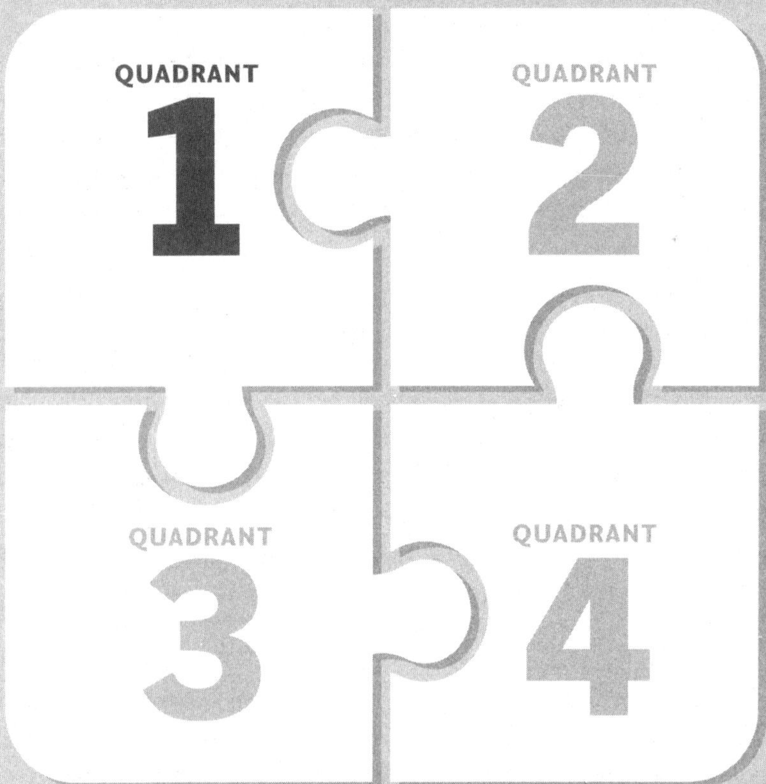

INFORMATICS

Welcome to the first part of your health ecosystem: INFORMATICS. This is where the numbers meet your story. It encompasses not only the clinical measurements that fill your medical chart—blood pressure readings, cholesterol levels, imaging results—but also the biographical details that rarely make it into any electronic health record: the childhood experiences, environmental exposures, relationship patterns, and life stressors that profoundly shape your well-being.

This is the quadrant in which medicine both succeeds brilliantly and fails spectacularly. A blood test can detect diabetes before you have any symptoms, potentially preventing devastating complications. Yet that same system might completely miss the facts that your blood sugar spikes started the month your mother with dementia moved in and your HbA1c level normalized after you addressed the caregiver stress driving your late-night eating patterns.

Understanding your INFORMATICS quadrant means becoming literate in the language of your own health data while recognizing that the most important health information often can't be measured. It's about knowing which numbers actually matter for your situation versus which ones create unnecessary anxiety. It's about ensuring that your complete story—not just your lab results—informs your care.

Most important, it's about recognizing that you are the bridge between the clinical data that doctors collect and the lived experience that creates the context of that data. When a patient tells me that their migraines started after they changed jobs, their joint pain flares during emotional stress, or their blood pressure readings vary dramatically depending on who's taking them, this biographical context transforms meaningless numbers into actionable intelligence.

In the following chapters, we'll explore how to navigate this complex relationship between objective measurements and subjective experience. You'll learn how to interpret your health data within the context of your unique situation, understand what crucial information might be missing entirely from your records, and become an active curator of your own health story.

By the end of this section, you'll have the tools to transform from a passive recipient of test results into an informed interpreter of your health information—someone who can see both the forest and the trees in your medical data.

Understanding Health Data: Its Value and Limitations

The promise of modern medicine is that data will provide answers. Test results will explain your symptoms. Screenings will catch problems early. Biomarkers will predict your future health. But here's what medicine rarely acknowledges: Data without context is just a set of numbers on a page. The same cholesterol level that's perfectly normal for one person may signal serious risk for another. The "abnormal" finding that sends you into a panic might be meaningless, while the most important factors affecting your health may never show up on any test.

Understanding medical data—what it can tell you, what it can't, and why you need human expertise to interpret it—is essential to becoming your own best advocate. I also want you to recognize the difference between population-based data and the reality of individual patients; I hope it will help you understand how your doctor makes decisions. This chapter explores the relationship between the numbers in your chart and the reality of your health.

Context Is Everything

Medical data is critical for making diagnostic decisions and treatment plans. High blood sugar readings and a hemoglobin A1C level over 6.5% are how doctors diagnose diabetes; follow-up lab tests are how we monitor whether treatment is keeping a patient's diabetes under control. However, the real value of data comes from putting it into context, that is, interpreting it and communicating it in a way that makes sense to the patient. This task is about more than looking at lab tests or X-ray reports; it requires a medical translator. When data is clearly communicated and free of medical jargon, patients can make informed choices. They can better quantify risk and assess the trade-offs inherent in every decision.

Even the most mundane blood tests need context. Take, for example, a patient whose LDL ("bad") cholesterol level is 122 mg/dL. Most commercial laboratories will flag this level as "high," even though it is entirely acceptable for a healthy thirty-year-old patient with no other cardiac risk factors. Yet the identical LDL reading for someone with existing heart disease is a significant concern requiring medical treatment.

My patient David exemplifies this principle. His LDL was 122 mg/dL, and his lipoprotein(a) level was elevated at 189 mg/dL. His father had died of a heart attack at age sixty-two. Generic advice (e.g., "keep exercising and eating healthy") wasn't going to be enough. When his coronary artery calcium scan revealed significant plaque accumulation in the arteries of his heart, his target LDL cholesterol level shifted dramatically. The LDL goal for patients with coronary heart disease is under 70 mg/dL. For very high-risk patients, it's under 55 mg/dL. This is based on evidence showing that this reduces cardiovascular events such as heart attacks and strokes. Given this context, David's LDL was too high. He needed more than a healthy lifestyle; he needed an evidence-based tool—a statin drug—to mitigate cardiovascular risk.

This principle of individualized risk stratification applies across all medical measurements. A blood pressure of 138/88 mmHg might be perfectly acceptable for an eighty-year-old with several chronic conditions, but it would raise concerns for a thirty-five-year-old, especially one with a family history of hypertension. The threshold for treatment is determined not by the number alone but by how that number relates to the patient's overall risk profile, age, medical history, and personal preferences.

In today's digital landscape, health information comes at us from all directions, often without proper context. Fear-inducing headlines about deadly viruses, new cancer warnings, and conflicting nutrition research flood our news feeds. One day carrots cause cancer; the next day they cure it. News outlets typically focus on grabbing your attention rather than providing the context needed to understand what new findings really mean for your health. A study showing that a 50 percent increased risk of something that affects 2 people per 100,000 sounds terrifying until you realize that it means 3 people per 100,000—still an extremely rare occurrence!

Meanwhile, patients often have access to their laboratory and imaging results through patient portals, sometimes before the ordering physician has had a chance to review, interpret, and communicate the findings. This immediate access, while empowering in theory, frequently leads to anxiety, fear, and late-night internet searches for self-diagnosis. A slightly elevated liver enzyme sends someone spiraling into worst-case scenarios, while a "borderline" result on a screening test triggers panic about diseases they may not even have.

This is precisely why you need a medical partner who can help you navigate your data thoughtfully. The same test result that might indicate serious concern in one patient could be completely normal for another, and distinguishing between these scenarios requires medical expertise, knowledge of your complete health picture, and an understanding of how different factors interact. Understanding how doctors approach and interpret this data can help you become a more informed participant in your own care.

How Doctors Make Decisions (and What Gets Lost in Translation)

A favorite expression I learned during residency was "Trust in God. Everyone else must bring data." This captures the way modern medicine tries to make decisions: by using the best available research rather than just going with hunches or tradition.

This approach, called evidence-based medicine (EBM), is why doctors today don't prescribe bloodletting for fevers or mercury for syphilis as they did a century ago. It's why we know that statins prevent heart attacks and why certain cancer treatments work. Medical science has gotten really good at figuring out what works for large groups of people.

But here's the catch: You're not a large group; you're one person with your own biology, life circumstances, and preferences. And sometimes what works "on average" doesn't work for you specifically.

Think of it as being like weather forecasting: When meteorologists say there's a 70 percent chance of rain, they're making a prediction based on hundreds of similar historical weather patterns. But that doesn't tell you whether it will rain on your picnic. You might be in the 30 percent who stay dry, or you might get caught in a downpour while the next town over stays sunny.

Medical research works similarly. Studies can tell us that a blood pressure medication works for seven out of ten people, but they can't predict whether you'll be one of the seven or one of the three who experience side effects instead of benefits.

When Medical Guidelines Collide: The Problem of Being Human

Randomized controlled trials tell us what works best on average for groups, but individual patients, especially patients confronting several medical conditions simultaneously, deviate from averages in important ways. Clinical practice guidelines typically focus on single diseases, creating challenges when someone has diabetes, heart failure, chronic kidney disease, and chronic obstructive pulmonary disease (COPD) all at once.

I remember when Paulette arrived at my office with a plastic shopping bag containing seventeen prescription medications. At seventy-six, she was managing several conditions, each requiring its own specialist and treatment regimen. "I can't do this anymore," she said, emptying the bottles onto my desk. "I take pills before breakfast, with breakfast, after breakfast, at lunch, before dinner, at bedtime—some with food, some without. My whole life revolves around these medications."

Each of Paulette's specialists followed their respective guidelines perfectly. Her endocrinologist aimed for an A1C level below 7%, her cardiologist optimized her heart failure medications, her pulmonologist managed her COPD exacerbations, and her nephrologist monitored her kidney function. But Paulette existed at the intersection of four evidence-based guidelines that, when combined, created an impossible treatment burden. The beta-blocker for her heart conflicted with her COPD management. Fluid restrictions for heart failure made it difficult to maintain the hydration recommended for her kidneys. Steroids for her breathing problems wreaked havoc on her glucose control.

"I don't know which doctor to listen to anymore," she confessed. "They all say different things, and when I tell one about side effects from another's medications, they just tell me to follow up with that specialist."

EBM failed Paulette because it was centered on diseases, not on Paulette herself. The art of medicine lies in marrying medical evidence with the patient in front of you, addressing their unique circumstances and personal preferences. Together, we simplified her medication regimen by accepting less aggressive targets in some areas and coordinating a team approach with her specialists. The result wasn't textbook perfection for any single condition, but it was a livable solution for the person sitting before me.

Why Good Medicine Often Lags Behind Good Science

Even when doctors have access to the latest research, medical practice often lags years or even decades behind evolving evidence. Thousands of new studies are published monthly, making it nearly impossible for practicing physicians to stay current with every development. Add to this the natural human tendency to stick with familiar approaches, and you have a recipe for medical time lag that can profoundly impact patient care.

Consider the ongoing story of menopause hormone therapy, a perfect example of how outdated medical thinking can persist long after the science has evolved. For decades, doctors advised women to avoid hormones after menopause, fearing an increased risk of developing breast cancer and heart disease. This belief was based on a flawed interpretation of the initial Women's Health Initiative study results in 2002.

When the data was revisited in the early 2010s, it became clear that the original conclusions had been overstated and misunderstood. The risks and benefits of hormone therapy are strongly influenced by age and timing, with more favorable outcomes when initiated in women younger than sixty or within ten years of menopause onset. By the time the messaging caught up to the data, a generation of women had been misled due to fear-based medical advice.

My patient Gilda was a classic victim of the gap between data and clinical practice standards. The fifty-eight-year-old retired school administrator had spent years bouncing between doctors for persistent hip pain and recurring urinary tract infections (UTIs). Her orthopedist attributed her hip pain to arthritis that was visible on X-rays, while her gynecologist treated each UTI as an isolated infection. When Gilda came to my office, frustrated and resigned to these issues being "part of getting older," I asked her questions no one had posed before: about vaginal dryness, sexual discomfort, and whether she'd been offered hormone therapy. Her gynecologist had dismissed hormone therapy due to her mother's breast cancer history—a decision based on outdated fears rather than current evidence.

Gilda's real problem was classic postmenopausal estrogen deficiency. Low estrogen levels weaken the pelvic floor muscles and urogenital tissues, creating her exact symptoms. I started her on vaginal estrogen cream and referred her to pelvic floor physical therapy. Within weeks, her UTIs disappeared and her hip pain, misattributed to arthritis, faded away.

The saddest part of that story? It can take generations for doctors to absorb new medical data and incorporate it into their clinical practice. In Gilda's case, even her gynecologist hadn't adopted the current evidence-based guidelines. Yet how would she have known how to advocate for herself? She trusted that her doctors were following the best available evidence, when in fact they were operating on outdated assumptions.

This disconnect between evolving science and clinical practice reveals a crucial truth: Having access to the right data isn't enough if the human elements of healthcare—communication, trust, and genuine listening—are missing. Gilda's years of suffering weren't caused by a lack of medical knowledge or sophisticated tests; they were caused by doctors who failed to ask the right questions, consider her complete picture, or challenge their own assumptions. The most advanced medical data in the world becomes meaningless without healthcare providers who can truly see and hear their patients.

This brings us to perhaps the most overlooked factor in all of medicine: the quality of the relationship between doctor and patient.

What Lab Tests Can't Measure: The Hidden Factors That Determine Your Health

In our data-obsessed healthcare system, we can measure inflammation down to the nanogram, sequence entire genomes, and track heart rhythms in real time. Patients track their steps, sleep, and grams of protein consumed. Yet medicine consistently fails to measure the factors that often matter most: the quality of trust between doctor and patient, how well treatments align with your personal values, and the complex web of relationships among your stress level, relationships, sleep, and physical symptoms.

We can quantify your cortisol level but not whether you feel heard during medical appointments. We can measure your cholesterol level but not how your work stress affects your eating patterns. We can sequence your DNA but not assess how your childhood experiences shape your health behaviors today. These invisible, interconnected factors frequently determine whether a treatment will succeed or fail—yet they rarely appear on any test or in any medical chart.

Trust: The Invisible Medicine That Makes Everything Else Work

Trust is the invisible infrastructure upon which all medical care is built. Listening, understanding, and honoring a patient's experience cannot be readily quantified, yet these human elements often determine whether a treatment succeeds or fails. While medical evidence is prioritized in research hierarchies, the relational factors that make medicine work are rarely measured at all. There is no lab test for the crucial human connection that facilitates healing.

Without trust, even the most sophisticated treatments become worthless. A patient who doesn't trust their doctor might nod politely during an appointment but never fill a prescription. They might agree to a treatment plan but abandon it at the first sign of side effects. They might withhold crucial information about symptoms or behaviors out of fear of judgment. In each case, perfectly good medical evidence becomes functionally useless when the human relationship fails.

Consider Lara, a sixty-four-year-old woman with diabetes who had cycled through three endocrinologists in four years. Each doctor had had access to the same evidence-based guidelines and prescribed similar medication regimens. Yet her blood glucose readings remained dangerously elevated, and her A1C level kept climbing despite multiple medication adjustments. When she came to my practice, I noticed her defensive posture and reluctance to make eye contact. Instead of immediately diving into her lab results, I asked about her experience living with diabetes, her daily routines, her challenges, her fears.

"No one's ever asked me that before," she said, finally looking up. Over the next three visits, she revealed that her previous doctor had made her feel ashamed about her weight and diet choices. As a result, she had never felt comfortable discussing her real struggles: avoiding exercise because of body shame and stress eating late at night when she felt overwhelmed. She assumed that any doctor would judge her, so she had simply stopped being honest about her behaviors. Once we established trust, and once she knew that I saw her as a whole person rather than a collection of failing metrics, everything changed. She became an engaged participant in her care. Her glucose control improved dramatically, not because I prescribed different medications but because I prescribed them within a relationship built on mutual respect and understanding.

James, a thirty-eight-year-old with severe hypertension, had a medical chart that read like a litany of provider frustration: "noncompliant," "difficult patient," "refuses to take medications as prescribed." When he finally landed in my office after an ER visit for dangerously high blood pressure, I could immediately sense his mistrust of the medical system. Instead of lecturing him about his cardiovascular risks, I asked what he thought was happening with his health.

"Nobody listens," he said, his arms crossed defensively. "They just want me to take pills that make me feel terrible." His concerns about medication side effects weren't irrational. One drug had affected his sexual function; another had made him so drowsy that he couldn't work effectively. Those weren't minor inconveniences; they were quality-of-life issues that previous doctors had dismissed. "Those are completely valid concerns," I told him, because they were. By listening, acknowledging his experiences, and offering him treatment options that addressed his worries, we slowly built enough trust for him to try a different medication regimen. His blood pressure became well controlled not by stronger medications but through a strong therapeutic alliance.

It's a low bar.

These cases illustrate how the invisible architecture of the patient-doctor relationship determines whether medical evidence will translate into improved health. This relational dimension explains why two patients with identical diagnoses and treatment plans often experience dramatically different outcomes. It also explains why evidence-based medicine, for all its scientific rigor, sometimes fails to deliver its promised benefits in real-world settings.

Without attention being paid to the human experience, even perfect data remains inert, like sophisticated software running on an outdated computer. The hardware may be flawless, but nothing happens without the right connections. Perhaps most important, it is within trusting therapeutic relationships that patients develop the confidence to participate in shared decision-making: weighing evidence against their personal values, preferences, and risk tolerance. The best medical decisions don't emerge when doctors simply download data and best practices to passive recipients; they happen when patients and doctors collaboratively interpret what that evidence *means* for this specific person's life. The relationship itself becomes medicine, often more powerful than any prescription or diagnostic test. Yet in our rush to optimize data and streamline care, we risk losing the human elements that make healing possible.

What's Worth It to You? Making Medical Decisions That Match Your Values

Central to the art of medicine is understanding each patient's unique tolerance for risk—a personal calculus as individual as their fingerprint. What one patient considers an acceptable medication side effect might be completely intolerable to another, and both perspectives are equally valid.

This is particularly significant in cancer care, in which doctors often default to recommending the most aggressive treatment protocols possible, assuming that patients will prioritize intensive cancer treatment at all costs. Yet, when fully educated on the risks and benefits of various treatments, many cancer patients may reasonably choose less aggressive approaches that offer a better quality of life, even if their length of survival isn't optimized.

I remember talking with my patient Rachel, a seventy-two-year-old artist with early-stage breast cancer, after her oncologist recommended the standard protocol: surgery, radiation, and five years of hormonal therapy. That approach offered the best statistical chance of preventing a recurrence, but Rachel was concerned about the cognitive side effects of hormonal therapy. As a painter whose identity and livelihood depended on her creative abilities, she valued her cognitive clarity above a reduction in recurrence risk.

"What good is living longer if I can't do the thing that makes me feel alive?" she asked. After considerable discussion about evidence, alternatives, and trade-offs, Rachel chose surgery and radiation but declined hormonal therapy. It wasn't "optimal" treatment according to the guidelines (and her oncologist expressed his displeasure with her decision!); however, it was optimal for her life and values.

My personal risk tolerance should never dictate the advice I give my patients. Instead, my responsibility is to arm my patients with clear, contextualized data about potential benefits and harms, help them understand how they apply to their specific situation, and support them in making decisions aligned with their own values and priorities.

The Web of Health: How Everything Connects to Everything Else

Medicine today faces another fundamental challenge: It struggles to capture the web of relationships that define how health works in real life. While medical research—studying this drug for that condition or measuring how this supplement affects that biomarker—excels at isolating variables, the human body operates as an integrated system in which everything influences everything else. Traditional medical research struggles to study these interconnections because they're difficult to control and measure. How do you design a randomized controlled trial that captures the relationship between someone's work stress, family dynamics, sleep quality, and digestive health? How do you isolate the effect of improved communication with a spouse on blood sugar control or measure the impact of meaningful work on immune function?

Yet these relationships often determine whether treatments succeed or fail. A patient's diabetes medication may work perfectly in clinical trials but fail in real life if chronic stress keeps the patient's cortisol level elevated, disrupting glucose metabolism. An antidepressant might show excellent efficacy in studies but provide little benefit if underlying sleep apnea continues to disrupt the brain chemistry the drug is trying to balance.

This doesn't diminish the value of rigorous medical data; lab results, imaging studies, and biomarkers remain essential to understanding your health. But it means that the most meaningful insights emerge when we view data within the context of your complete health ecosystem. Your cholesterol number becomes more informative when we consider it alongside your stress patterns, sleep quality, family history, and current life circumstances. Your inflammatory markers tell a richer story when viewed in relation to your gut health, exercise habits, emotional state, and environmental exposures.

The goal isn't to make your definition of health more complicated but to make it more complete. As you begin to map your own health ecosystem in the coming chapters, pay attention not just to individual symptoms or measurements but to the patterns and relationships among them. The most profound improvements in health often come not from optimizing isolated factors but from understanding and nurturing the connections between them.

The Data Doctors Collect and Why It Matters

Robert arrived at my office clutching a folder of lab results, his face a mixture of frustration and concern. "Everything's normal," he said, sliding the papers across my desk. "Every test is in range. So why do I feel like I'm walking through quicksand every day?" His comprehensive bloodwork, ordered by three different specialists over six months, showed textbook results. His complete blood count, metabolic panel, thyroid function, vitamin levels: All were within normal ranges. Yet his crushing fatigue, brain fog, and joint pain had only worsened. "My rheumatologist said maybe it's just stress," he explained. "My cardiologist suggested I exercise more. My neurologist ordered an MRI that showed nothing concerning. I'm starting to think it's all in my head." Robert's experience highlights a fundamental truth about medical data: It can tell us many things but rarely everything.

QUICK REFERENCE
The Problem with "Normal" Lab Values

- "Normal" lab values represent population averages, not individual optimals.
- You can have "normal" lab values and still feel unwell.
- You can have "abnormal" lab values and feel perfectly fine.
- Test results represent snapshots in time that require clinical context to be appropriately interpreted.
- Many important health factors don't show up on standard tests.

Decoding the Patient Chart

Let's talk about the patient chart, also known as your electronic health record, or EHR. As discussed in chapter 1, an EHR is intended to be a repository of patient data and information. At its best, it serves as a comprehensive digital version of a patient's medical history, including lab results, imaging reports, medication lists, allergies, past diagnoses, and physician notes. It ensures that important medical data is readily available, reducing the risk of errors, unnecessary tests, and fragmented care across different providers.

The truth is that EHRs serve more as billing and compliance tools than as a home for patient-centered recordkeeping and decision-making. Unlike in many other developed countries, there is no centralized EHR system in the United States. Each healthcare system, hospital network, and sometimes individual practice maintains its own electronic records. This means that you likely have a distinct, and often disparate and incomplete, digital footprint in different medical places.

It's no wonder that patients have taken data collecting into their own hands; they are charting themselves. It's partly why so many people, most of whom would describe themselves as "health conscious," are walking around with step counters, heart monitors, sleep trackers, Oura rings, and continuous glucose monitors. Patients assume that if their Oura ring says they are sleeping well and their step counter says they're stepping, they are okay. But where is the integration of this medical data into how we feel? Who is the owner of this bloodwork or that enlarged liver or leaky heart valve? How can your symptoms be heard through the morass of informatics?

While understanding how medical information is stored and shared is important, let's step back and examine what data doctors truly need from you during an appointment—and why some of the most crucial information never makes it into any electronic system.

What Data Is Your Doctor Looking For?

You are sitting in a doctor's exam room or office, waiting to be seen. Most people are accustomed to filling out forms in advance of the appointment, only to be asked the same questions again in the office. So what data and information are doctors seeking when they see you? Is there a more accurate dataset that your doctor might glean from you or that you might give your doctor at the outset of your visit? What data do they really need to provide medical advice?

The data primary care doctors need and collect at a new-patient visit includes your comprehensive medical history: all known past and present medical conditions, both acute and chronic. Conditions such as hypertension, diabetes, asthma, thyroid disease, autoimmune disorders, and cancer are key factors that warrant further testing and treatment.

Your surgical history is another crucial component. Any past surgeries, from routine procedures such as an appendectomy to more complex operations such as open-heart surgery or joint replacements, provide insight into potential complications, lingering symptoms, or the need for follow-up care. Your doctor will also ask about hospitalizations, even if they were for nonsurgical reasons. A history of hospitalization for pneumonia, kidney infections, or mental health crises provides important context for understanding your current health concerns.

Your complete medical history provides context that isolated data points cannot. It's the narrative thread that helps make sense of otherwise disconnected numbers and images.

Your family history plays a vital role in identifying genetic risk factors. Your doctor will ask about conditions including heart disease, stroke, cancer, diabetes, osteoporosis, and mental health disorders in your immediate family. A history of early-onset heart disease (such as a parent who had a heart attack before age fifty-five) signals a need for more aggressive cardiovascular risk assessment. A strong family history of colon cancer may mean that screening should begin earlier than the standard guideline of age forty-five. Unfortunately, family history takes us only so far. With breast cancer, for instance, the public perception focuses heavily on genetic mutations, specifically BRCA1 and BRCA2. These mutations significantly increase the risk of developing certain cancers, but they account for only 5 to 10 percent of breast cancers. The reality? About 85 percent of breast cancers occur in women with no family history. This doesn't mean that family history isn't important; it is. Having a first-degree relative who had breast cancer nearly doubles your risk. But the *absence* of a family history doesn't mean you're in the clear, and the presence of a strong family history doesn't mean that you're destined to get it.

Understanding this helps patients make more informed decisions about genetic testing and screening without succumbing to either false reassurances or unnecessary fear.

The Physical Examination: What Your Body Reveals

Beyond gathering your medical history, the physical exam provides real-time data about your body's current state. Doctors listen to your heart and lungs, examine your abdomen, check for enlarged lymph nodes, and assess for masses, rashes, and skeletal asymmetries. They assess various body systems based on your age, symptoms, and concerns.

Perhaps most important, the physical exam creates a moment of genuine connection, a time when your doctor is fully present with you, using all their senses and training to understand what's happening in your body. This hands-on assessment often reveals subtle findings that no questionnaire or computer screen can capture, while building the trust essential for effective healthcare. Beyond these measurable findings, the physical exam allows me to observe subtle cues that reveal crucial information about my patients' well-being. The way someone sits, for example, hunched forward with protective posturing, often tells me more about their pain level than their verbal description does. A patient's gait as they walk to the exam room can reveal neurological concerns before any formal testing is done. The color of their skin, the quality of their breathing, and their overall energy level provide immediate insights into illness severity that no virtual visit can capture.

Vital Signs: The Numbers That Track Your Basic Functions

Vital signs include blood pressure, heart rate, respiratory rate, temperature, height, weight, and body mass index (BMI). When I take a patient's vital signs, I'm gathering a set of fundamental measurements that can reveal both immediate concerns and long-term patterns. These aren't just numbers; they're reflections of your intricate bodily systems' reactions to your combination of age, genetics, diet, fitness, and hormonal status.

Consider Maria, who came to my office complaining of headaches. Her blood pressure reading of 168/95 mmHg immediately told me something important: that her arteries were under significant strain. But it also told a more interesting story. Maria hadn't slept in days due to an ill child. She'd been living on coffee and comfort food. Her high blood pressure wasn't just a medical fact; it reflected her life circumstances.

The Special Case of Weight and BMI: Beyond the Number on the Scale

A patient's weight and BMI only tell one part of their metabolic story. Of course, significant changes in weight can indicate important shifts in metabolic health, and excess adipose tissue is known to create inflammation and hormonal disruption. But weight is one data point among many, and it's often not the most important one. This vital sign alone is one of the most common reasons people avoid doctors.

For example, my patient Sophia had a BMI that placed her in the "overweight" category. Her mother put her on a strict diet when she was twelve years old. Doctors had counseled her to lose weight since she was in high school. Unsurprisingly, the constant focus on the number on the scale had taken a toll on her sense of self-worth. When she came to see me as a new patient in her sixties, she expected to hear the same refrain.

But when I looked at her complete health picture, I saw something different. Her blood pressure was a normal 118/76. Her cholesterol profile was excellent—optimal LDL, high HDL, and normal triglycerides. Her A1C and fasting glucose were in perfect ranges. She exercised four days a week, ate a primarily plant-based diet rich in whole foods, and slept well. By every measure except BMI, Sophia was metabolically healthy. The number on the scale told me almost nothing about the actual state of her metabolic health.

Recent data suggests that over 88 percent of American adults have some degree of metabolic dysfunction. Yet medical professionals often focus exclusively on weight and BMI, metrics that can be profoundly misleading. Someone can have a "normal" BMI and terrible metabolic health if they're sedentary, eat poorly, or carry most of their fat around their organs. Conversely, someone like Sophia can have a higher BMI and be remarkably healthy if they're muscular, active, and carry their weight in metabolically safer locations.

The real story of metabolic health happens beneath the surface, in how your body processes energy, responds to food, manages stress, and regulates inflammation. These processes determine whether you'll develop diabetes, heart disease, fatty liver disease, and countless other conditions—regardless of what you weigh.

As you think about your own vital signs, remember that they exist in the context of your life. To understand how metabolically healthy you are, the question isn't "What do you weigh?" but rather "How effectively does your body regulate blood sugar, respond to insulin, manage inflammation, and maintain energy throughout the day?"

For Sophia, understanding this distinction was transformative. She stopped trying to shrink her body and started focusing on keeping it strong, well-rested, and metabolically flexible. Her labs remained excellent. Her energy stayed consistent. And the mental space she'd spent worrying about her weight became available for everything else in her life that actually mattered.

Context Matters for All Vital Signs

Blood pressure might spike due to stress or insomnia; it can drop due to dehydration, illness, or an overactive vagus nerve. I've seen patients whose blood pressure is perfectly controlled at home but spikes in my office—"white coat hypertension" driven purely by medical anxiety. Certain medications such as Advil and Motrin elevate blood pressure; some eye drops used to treat glaucoma can lower it.

Heart rate tends to dip when you are sleeping; it also reflects your fitness level, stress hormone axis, caffeine and alcohol consumption, hydration status, and alertness. A marathon runner might have a resting heart rate in the 40s that would alarm us in someone sedentary. Grief, excitement, or the third cup of coffee can all send your heart rate climbing.

Respiratory rate can reveal anxiety as much as lung function. A patient sitting in my office breathing rapidly at 24 breaths per minute might be having a panic attack, dealing with pneumonia, or experiencing heart failure. The number alone doesn't tell me which—I need the rest of the story.

Temperature isn't just about infection; it follows daily cycles and can reflect thyroid function and overall endocrine status. Some people run consistently cool or warm. I've learned to ask patients, "What's normal for you?" rather than assuming 98.6°F is everyone's baseline.

Weight fluctuates with variations in your hydration, hormone levels, salt intake, and countless other factors. That five-pound gain over a weekend might reflect the salty restaurant meal and interrupted sleep, not a fundamental change in your body composition.

While vital signs provide immediate insights into your body's current state, blood tests offer a window into your internal environment, revealing processes that are invisible to the naked eye but equally dependent on context for meaningful interpretation.

Blood Tests: Windows into Your Internal Environment

Blood work reveals important elements of your health. It reveals infections, anemia, dehydration, and menopause. Specific substances in your blood, such as glucose and potassium, show us how your major organ systems, such as your heart, liver and kidneys, are performing. Blood work tells us how well you eliminate bodily waste and how well your hormonal systems are functioning. It can raise alarm bells for substance abuse, infection, and certain types of cancer. It can help us assess your risk of developing certain cancers before you get sick. It can help us understand your risk of developing atherosclerosis before you have a heart attack or stroke. It can detect genetic disorders, autoimmune diseases, and hidden inflammation.

However, interpreting blood work requires context. Despite patients' temptations to plug their lab results into Google or ChatGPT in order to deem themselves "healthy" or to make a definitive self-diagnosis, lab results in a vacuum can be misleading. They also don't tell a complete story. Take, for example, the question of metabolic health. In my practice, I see the earliest signs of metabolic dysfunction long before lab values show prediabetes or diabetes. Patients describe energy crashes in the afternoon, feeling shaky if they skip meals, difficulty concentrating after eating, or that peculiar "wired but tired" sensation. Sleep disruption is enormous. Many people wake between 2 and 4 a.m. as their body releases stress hormones to compensate for blood sugar dips during the night. Others have lost touch with normal hunger and fullness cues entirely, eating either nothing until they're ravenous or continuing until they're uncomfortably stuffed. These subjective experiences matter as much as any lab value because they reflect what's happening at the cellular level. When your body struggles to regulate blood sugar effectively, you feel it in your energy, your mood, your sleep, and your relationship with food—often years before a doctor diagnoses you with anything.

Another limitation of blood work is that it only captures a single moment in time. It tells us how your body was functioning when blood spilled out of your arm into a test tube. The numbers can fluctuate depending on the time of day, when and what you last ate, and whether or not you recently had an illness, surgery, infection, or vaccine dose. We use ranges to decide what numbers are normal, but you can have a number outside the normal range and be healthy or a number in the normal range and be unwell.

When you receive lab results from your doctor, you'll typically see a collection of tests with numbers and reference ranges. Understanding what these tests measure can help you become a more informed participant in your healthcare.

QUICK REFERENCE
Understanding Common Lab Tests

Complete Blood Count (CBC)

This foundational test evaluates your blood cells and provides critical information about your overall health.

- **Red blood cell (RBC) count:** The number of oxygen-carrying cells in your blood. A low number may indicate anemia, while a high number can suggest dehydration or certain blood disorders.
- **Hemoglobin (Hgb):** The protein in red blood cells that carries oxygen. A low level can indicate anemia, blood loss, or nutritional deficiencies, while a high level might suggest dehydration, smoking, or lung disease.
- **Hematocrit (Hct):** The percentage of your blood volume occupied by red blood cells. This provides information similar to hemoglobin but from a different angle.
- **White blood cell (WBC) count:** The number of immune cells in your blood. An elevated level often indicates infection or inflammation, while a low level might suggest bone marrow problems or certain medications.
- **Platelet count:** Cell fragments that help blood clot. A low count may increase bleeding risk, while a high count can sometimes indicate inflammation or a bone marrow disorder.

Comprehensive Metabolic Panel (CMP)

This panel examines your organ function and metabolic health through fourteen different measurements.

- **Glucose:** Your blood sugar level. A high level may indicate diabetes or prediabetes, while a low level could suggest hypoglycemia.
- **Electrolytes (sodium, potassium, chloride, bicarbonate):** Minerals that are crucial for nerve function, muscle contraction, and maintaining proper bodily pH. Imbalances can affect heart rhythm, muscle function, and more.
- **Calcium:** Essential for bone health, muscle function, and nerve signaling. An abnormal level may indicate hormone problems, vitamin D deficiency, or kidney issues.
- **Kidney function (BUN, creatinine):** Waste products that reflect how well your kidneys are filtering your blood. Elevated levels suggest decreased kidney function.
- **Liver function (AST, ALT, ALP, bilirubin, albumin, total protein):** Enzymes and proteins that indicate liver health. Elevation may suggest liver inflammation, medication effects, or liver disease.

Lipid Panel

This panel evaluates your cardiovascular risk by measuring fat molecules in your blood.

- **Total cholesterol:** The sum of all cholesterol in your blood. While important, this number alone doesn't tell the complete story of heart risk.
- **HDL cholesterol:** Often called "good" cholesterol because it helps remove other forms of cholesterol from your bloodstream. A higher level is generally protective.
- **LDL cholesterol:** Often called "bad" cholesterol because it can build up in artery walls. A lower level is typically better for heart health.
- **Triglycerides:** Another type of fat in your blood. An elevated level is associated with heart disease, diabetes, and other conditions.

Thyroid Function Tests

These tests assess how well your thyroid gland is working.

- **Thyroid-stimulating hormone (TSH):** Produced by the pituitary gland to regulate the thyroid. A high level often indicates an underactive thyroid (hypothyroidism), while a low level suggests an overactive thyroid (hyperthyroidism).

- **Free T4 and free T3:** Actual thyroid hormones. Their values help clarify thyroid function, especially when TSH is abnormal.

Hemoglobin A1C Test

This test measures your average blood sugar level over the previous two to three months.

- A normal A1C is below 5.7%.
- Prediabetes ranges from 5.7% to 6.4%.
- Diabetes is diagnosed at 6.5% or higher.

Unlike a single glucose reading, A1C gives a longer-term picture of blood sugar control.

Vitamin Levels

Common vitamin tests include:

- **Vitamin D:** Essential for bone health, immune function, and more. Deficiency is surprisingly common, even in sunny climates.
- **Vitamin B12:** Crucial for nerve function and blood cell formation. A low level can cause anemia and neurological problems.
- **Folate (vitamin B9):** Important for promoting cell division and preventing certain birth defects. Deficiency can lead to a specific type of anemia.

Iron Levels

These tests assess iron status and help diagnose various types of anemia.

- **Ferritin:** Stored iron. A low level indicates iron deficiency, while a high level might suggest iron overload or inflammation.
- **Iron and TIBC (total iron binding capacity):** Together, these measurements help distinguish among different types of anemia.
- **Transferrin saturation:** Calculated from iron and TIBC, this percentage indicates how much iron is available for use.

Inflammation Markers

These tests are nonspecific markers of inflammation.

- **C-reactive protein (CRP):** This can indicate an infection, an inflammatory process, or autoimmune disease, among other conditions. A high-sensitivity CRP (hs-CRP) test can also help assess cardiovascular risk.

- **Sedimentation rate (ESR):** Similar to the CRP, this measures how quickly red blood cells settle at the bottom of a test tube, which indirectly indicates the amount of inflammation in the body.

Tests of cardiovascular risk

- **Lipoprotein (a) or Lp(a):** This is a test for a specific type of low-density lipoprotein (LDL) cholesterol, often called "bad" cholesterol, which is genetically determined. High levels of Lp(a) are a significant risk factor for heart attack, stroke, and other cardiovascular diseases.
- **Apolipoprotein B or ApoB:** This measures the number of apolipoprotein B particles in your blood, which are the main protein components of LDL cholesterol particles. High ApoB levels are a strong indicator of cardiovascular risk because more particles mean more "bad" cholesterol.

Remember that lab values must always be interpreted in the context of your overall health, symptoms, and medical history. A number that's slightly outside the "normal" range doesn't necessarily indicate disease; conversely, you can have symptoms despite having "normal" results. The real challenge lies in recognizing the utility and unintended consequences of medical testing.

Questions That Data Can and Cannot Answer

I call them "common diagnostic challenges"—the routine complaints that patients bring to my office. It might be exhaustion, mood swings, memory issues, or worries about inflammation, but they have one thing in common: Patients usually want a "test" to figure out exactly what is going on.

"I Just Need Some Tests": When Normal Lab Results Don't Tell the Whole Story

"I don't feel well, I just need some labs," begins a typical message from a patient. Whether it's fatigue, brain fog, or memory concerns, patients understandably want answers, preferably in the form of a number to measure and fix.

Sarah, a forty-nine-year-old executive, was convinced that she had some underlying disease that was causing her exhaustion and brain fog. "I need a brain MRI," she messaged me. "My mother had Alzheimer's, and I'm terrified I'm heading down the same path." She also requested the APOE4 genetic test, having read online that it could predict her risk of developing Alzheimer's. She was certain that one of those tests would either confirm her fears or put them to rest. I explained to her that having the APOE4 allele does not guarantee the development of Alzheimer's. Conversely, many people with Alzheimer's do not have the APOE4 allele. In other words, screening for Alzheimer's is much more complicated than doing a single test. A positive test could generate unnecessary fear in a patient whose cognitive symptoms could be explained by other factors.

Given these limitations of genetic testing, we decided to start with basic lab work. Everything came back normal—not a single value out of range—yet she could barely get through her workday without multiple cups of coffee and was increasingly forgetting names and losing her train of thought. When I examined her case more thoroughly, I discovered what her brain MRI and genetic test never would have shown. It wasn't until our in-person visit, when we spent time discussing her routines, that the picture became clear: She was answering emails until midnight, waking to check her phone at 4:00 a.m., skipping meals regularly, and carrying the emotional burden of a difficult workplace transition. Her "brain fog" worsened during her most stressful weeks, and her energy crashed every afternoon when her blood sugar level plummeted due to her irregular eating.

The standard fatigue workup (complete blood count, thyroid tests, vitamin B12 and iron levels) can identify common, treatable causes. But here's what many patients don't realize: Symptoms such as fatigue and cognitive issues are often the result of factors that no blood test can measure. The most important diagnostic tool in cases like Sarah's wasn't sophisticated testing; it was our conversation about her life, habits, and stressors. Within months of addressing her sleep hygiene, meal timing, and work boundaries, both her energy and her cognitive clarity returned to normal.

Sarah's story illustrates a crucial principle: The brain and body are exquisitely sensitive to lifestyle factors. Memory, focus, and energy depend on proper sleep, nutrition, stress management, and emotional well-being. Sometimes the most valuable intervention isn't a test result but a thorough examination of how you're living.

Am I in Perimenopause? The Art of Treating the Patient, Not the Test Result

"I need my hormones checked," declared Melissa, a forty-seven-year-old who had been experiencing irregular periods, mood swings, night sweats, and brain fog for the past year. "I've read everything online about perimenopause, and I'm sure that's what's happening. Can't you just check my estrogen and progesterone levels?" she asked, frustrated when I suggested that we might not need extensive lab work.

Melissa was right about her symptoms suggesting perimenopause, the transition period before menopause when ovarian function begins to decline. What many patients don't realize is that checking estrogen, progesterone, and FSH levels—the female reproductive hormones that change during perimenopause—typically is of limited diagnostic value. These hormone levels fluctuate dramatically during perimenopause, sometimes from day to day or even from hour to hour. A blood test simply tells us where the hormones are at the exact moment of the blood draw. A woman might have a normal estrogen level in the morning that plummets by evening, triggering night sweats. Or her FSH might be normal one week and elevated the next as her body tries to stimulate her ovaries. Furthermore, many women continue to have regular cycles with normal hormone levels while experiencing classic perimenopausal symptoms. Others might have wildly abnormal hormone values but feel fine.

Perimenopause is primarily a clinical diagnosis, made based on age, menstrual history, and symptom pattern. Similarly, menopause itself, defined as going twelve consecutive months without a period, doesn't require blood tests to confirm, though they may be helpful in ambiguous cases.

After discussing Melissa's symptoms in detail, I explained that her pattern of irregular periods, night sweats, mood changes, and brain fog at age forty-seven strongly suggested perimenopause, regardless of what any single hormone test might show. Instead of focusing on testing, we discussed treatment options to manage her symptoms, including lifestyle modifications, low-dose birth control pills, and other targeted therapies.

Melissa left with a treatment plan rather than a lab blood draw slip and reported significant improvement at her follow-up visit three months later. The lesson? Sometimes the most valuable diagnostic tool isn't a sophisticated test but a thorough conversation about symptoms in the context of a person's age and life stage.

"My Inflammation Is High": When Numbers Mislead

"My CRP is elevated. I must have dangerous inflammation!" This is a refrain I hear increasingly often as patients become more aware of inflammatory markers such as C-reactive protein (CRP).

The wellness industry and social media have turned inflammation into a bogeyman, a nebulous enemy to be fought with special diets, supplements, and detox regimens. And while chronic inflammation is indeed associated with numerous health problems from heart disease to autoimmune conditions, interpreting inflammatory markers requires significant context. Carlos came to me worried after an ER visit for a kidney stone revealed that his CRP level was elevated at 32 mg/L (normal is under 3 mg/L). The ER doctor had mentioned it in passing, and Carlos had immediately researched online, finding concerning connections between elevated CRP and heart disease, cancer, and autoimmune disorders. What he didn't read in his online searching, and what the ER doctor had failed to explain, is that the CRP level rises in response to any inflammation in the body. His kidney stone alone would cause significant CRP elevation. The fever he'd experienced would raise it further. Even the stress of the ER visit itself could contribute.

The CRP test is a perfect example of a test that requires context and clinical expertise and judgment. It can signal anything from rheumatoid arthritis to cancer to an infected fingernail to seasonal allergies to metabolic inefficiency to diabetes. In a vacuum, it is distinctly unhelpful. Importantly, CRP doesn't typically reflect mechanical inflammation such as osteoarthritis or an aching back after sitting on a long car ride. It also isn't always improved by the wellness industry's anti-inflammatory diets. Sure, antioxidant foods such as blueberries, avocado, and salmon are anti-inflammatory on a cellular level, but if your CRP is elevated because of appendicitis or breast cancer, no amount of blueberries and avocados will address the underlying cause.

After ruling out serious causes for Carlos's elevated CRP, I explained that the value would likely normalize within a week as his kidney stone resolved.

The Harms of Overtesting: Just Because You Can Doesn't Mean You Should

Medical imaging and specialized testing serve crucial roles when used appropriately. X-rays excel at revealing broken bones and lung infections. MRIs provide detailed images of soft tissues, making them invaluable for diagnosing brain injuries, torn ligaments, and spinal problems. CT scans can identify internal bleeding or detect tumors with precision. DEXA scans accurately measure bone density to diagnose osteoporosis. When ordered for specific medical concerns by trained physicians, these tests save lives and guide treatment decisions. But problems arise when these powerful diagnostic tools are misused as general screening methods or marketed directly to consumers as comprehensive health assessments. Two concerning trends have emerged: full-body MRIs promoted as preventive medicine and single blood tests promising to detect dozens of cancers simultaneously. Both represent the wellness industry's attempt to monetize our legitimate desire for health security, often creating more anxiety than answers.

Full-Body MRIs: The Illusion of Control

Scroll through Instagram or TikTok, and you'll likely encounter celebrities and wellness influencers touting full-body MRI scans as the ultimate in preventive healthcare. The companies that do them, often partnering with social media personalities, claim that their scans offer early detection of medical problems and peace of mind. But these expensive scans, typically costing $1,000 to $2,500 out of pocket, create more anxiety than answers. Up to 40 percent of people getting these scans will have "findings" that require follow-up testing, yet fewer than 1 percent will have clinically significant discoveries that will actually change their health outcomes. But the companies profit whether the results help you or not.

A full-body MRI shows incredibly detailed images of your organs, tissues, and blood vessels from head to toe. The problem? It shows everything, including countless normal variations, benign cysts, old injuries, and anatomical quirks that exist in most healthy people. A radiologist might report "multiple small liver lesions," "bilateral renal cysts," or "scattered white matter changes in the brain." To an untrained eye, these findings sound terrifying. They're often meaningless. The danger lies in what happens next. Each "incidental finding" typically requires follow-up testing, additional scans, blood work, sometimes even biopsies, to rule out serious disease. This cascade of testing creates anxiety, expense, and sometimes real harm due to unnecessary procedures being done.

I hope that someday our medical technology will be advanced enough that a full-body MRI can detect things that are worrisome and not detect things that aren't worrisome. I hope that someday MRIs will be able to capture the functional nuances of our organ systems and become effective, affordable screening tools. But we aren't there yet. Using a full-body MRI to assess our health is akin to scrolling through a person's Instagram feed to understand who they really are. Those carefully curated images give us lots of information, vacation destinations, aesthetic preferences, glimpses of social life, but there's no context to interpret what we're seeing, nor is it necessarily the data we need to judge what's truly happening in someone's life. We don't see the anxiety behind the perfect selfie, the financial stress that made taking that vacation a stretch, or the loneliness that prompted those social gathering posts. Similarly, an MRI might show a small cyst or unusual tissue density without revealing whether it's clinically significant, how long it's been there, or how it relates to your symptoms. Sometimes the most important information, such as the Instagrammer's authentic relationships or daily struggles, isn't captured in the image at all.

My best advice? Seek out a physician who will assess your whole health, not just a snapshot of your body parts, and make evidence-based recommendations for screening based on your age, risk factors, and medical history. There's no substitute for the personalized approach.

Galleri Testing: The Allure of a Single Test for Cancer

"My friend was just diagnosed with stage four pancreatic cancer," explained James, a healthy forty-five-year-old with no concerning symptoms or family history. "I want to get the Galleri test I saw advertised online that can detect over fifty types of cancer with a blood draw." The Galleri test, a blood test that claims to detect cancer-specific DNA fragments circulating in your bloodstream, seems like the perfect solution: simple, noninvasive, and comprehensive. The marketing promises early detection of dozens of cancer types that traditional screening often misses, including pancreatic, ovarian, and lung cancers. At around $950 out of pocket (insurance typically doesn't cover it), it's positioned as a premium health investment for those who can afford it.

But the reality is more complex than the advertising suggests. While the test can identify some cancers, it also produces false positives that lead to unnecessary anxiety and expensive follow-up testing. More concerning, it can miss early-stage cancers precisely when detection would be most valuable, while sometimes identifying advanced cancers that might have been caught through symptoms anyway. The test performs best on cancers we already screen for effectively, such as colorectal cancer, making its added value questionable. Perhaps most important, we don't yet know whether finding cancers through a Galleri test improves patient outcomes compared to standard screening methods. Early detection helps only if it leads to better treatment results, and that data simply doesn't exist yet. At this moment, tests such as the Galleri test can offer only expensive and imperfect reassurance to people who can afford them, while potentially creating more problems than they solve. The better way to screen for cancer? Following evidence-based recommendations for cancer screening.

QUICK REFERENCE
Recommended Core Cancer Screenings Based on Age

AGE-BASED CANCER SCREENING RECOMMENDATIONS

Ages 18 to 39

- **Cervical cancer:** Pap smear every three years starting at age twenty-one; after age thirty, you can opt for a Pap test every three years, HPV testing alone every five years, or cotesting for both every five years.
- **Skin cancer:** Annual skin checks for those with risk factors (fair skin, history of sunburns, family history).
- **Testicular cancer (men):** Self-exams encouraged; clinical exam as part of a routine physical.

Ages 40 to 49

- **Breast cancer:** Annual or biennial mammograms starting at age forty (the exact timing depends on personal risk factors and preference).
- **Cervical cancer:** Continue screening as above.
- **Colorectal cancer:** Begin screening at age forty-five with colonoscopy, fecal immunochemical (FIT) test, or other options.
- **Prostate cancer (men):** Discuss prostate-specific antigen (PSA) testing with your doctor starting at age forty-five to fifty, earlier for high-risk groups.
- **Skin cancer:** Annual skin checks, especially for those with risk factors.

Ages 50 to 64

- **Breast cancer:** Annual or biennial mammograms.
- **Cervical cancer:** Screening until age sixty-five.
- **Colorectal cancer:** Screening via colonoscopy every ten years, annual FIT test, or other approved methods.
- **Lung cancer:** Annual low-dose CT scan for current or former heavy smokers (twenty-plus packs per year history, quit within past fifteen years).
- **Prostate cancer (men):** PSA testing based on decisions made with a doctor.
- **Skin cancer:** Annual skin checks.

Ages 65+

- **Breast cancer:** Continue mammograms based on overall health and life expectancy.
- **Cervical cancer:** Can discontinue after age sixty-five with adequate prior negative screenings.
- **Colorectal cancer:** Continue until age seventy-five, then individualized decisions.
- **Lung cancer:** Continue annual screening if criteria are met and the patient is in good health.
- **Prostate cancer (men):** Individualized approach based on health status and life expectancy.

It's important to remember that these are general guidelines. Your specific screening plan should be personalized based on your family history, personal medical history, lifestyle factors, and other risk factors. Cancer isn't a single disease but a diverse collection of conditions with different risk factors and optimal screening approaches.

Genetic Testing: Your DNA Isn't Your Destiny

When patients request genetic testing, they usually arrive with one of two dangerous assumptions. Either they believe that having a genetic variant guarantees that they'll develop a disease, or they think that not having one means that they're completely safe. Both beliefs miss how genetics actually works.

"I have the MTHFR gene variant," Vanessa, a thirty-five-year-old, told me after ordering a direct-to-consumer genetic test. "The internet says I will get blood clots, heart disease, and pregnancy complications. I think I need blood-thinning medication." Meanwhile, Jason, a forty-two-year-old with a strong family history of heart disease, had the opposite reaction: "My genetic test was negative for cardiac risk genes, so I don't need to worry about my cholesterol or blood pressure anymore." Both patients had fallen into the trap of "genetic determinism," the mistaken belief that DNA controls destiny. The reality is far more hopeful: Your genes are not your fate. Think of DNA as providing the architectural plans for a house, but whether that house is actually built depends on countless other factors: the weather, the available materials, the skill of the workers, and how well the foundation is constructed.

The most compelling evidence comes from identical twin studies. These twins share exactly the same DNA, yet they often develop completely different health conditions as they age. One twin develops diabetes, while the other stays metabolically healthy. One gets Alzheimer's disease, while the other remains sharp into their nineties. The difference? Years of different environments, stress levels, diets, relationships, and lifestyle choices that influence how their identical genes are expressed.

Most genetic tests have limited predictive power because they cannot measure important factors that turn genetic predispositions into disease. For example, sleep, stress, systemic inflammation, certain lifestyle factors and environmental exposures play a role in determining who gets sick. There is no blood test to date that can measure the complex interplay between genetics and environmental factors. Therefore, genetic testing only makes sense when there is a clear family pattern of a disease that is known to be hereditary and when the results would change your behavior and/or your medical care plan.

How to Be Your Own Data Detective

How can you become a more informed participant in your own healthcare data collection? Here are some strategies to help you navigate the complex world of medical testing.

- **Ask why.** Before agreeing to any test, ask your doctor what specific question the test is designed to answer. Is it screening for a particular condition? Monitoring a known issue? Ruling out a specific concern?
- **Understand your "normal."** Laboratory reference ranges aren't one-size-fits-all. They are statistical averages derived from large populations, not absolute definitions of "healthy" versus "unhealthy." Understanding this distinction can prevent unnecessary anxiety and help you advocate for appropriate care.
- **Know your personal baseline.** Some people naturally run higher or lower than the statistical average for certain values. Take my patient Merrill, who has had slightly elevated liver enzymes her entire adult life. She takes no medications that would affect these values, and she has no symptoms. Various specialists have evaluated her for common and esoteric reasons for liver problems. She even had a liver biopsy that was normal. Yet every new doctor who sees her labs for the first time orders urgent follow-up tests and expresses concern. Merrill has learned to tell new providers up front, "My ALT has been sixty-five for fifteen years, it's been thoroughly investigated, and it's normal for me."
- **Consider the context of "abnormal."** A value slightly outside the reference range may be perfectly normal for you, especially if it's been consistent over time and you have no symptoms. Conversely, a significant change within the "normal" range might be more concerning than a stable "abnormal" result. If your creatinine (kidney function marker) suddenly jumps from 0.8 to 1.1 mg/dL—both technically normal—that 38 percent increase might warrant more attention than someone whose creatinine has been stable at 1.3 mg/dL for years.
- **Ask the right questions.** When facing an "abnormal" result, ask your doctor:

  "How far outside normal is this, and is that significant?"

"Is this a new change for me, or has it been consistent?"
"Given my symptoms and health history, should I be concerned?"
"Do we need to investigate this, or should we just monitor it?"

- **Keep your own records.** Track your key numbers over time and take this history to new providers. A simple note saying "My cholesterol runs high (usually around 240 mg/dL), but my ratios are good and it's been stable for ten years" can prevent unnecessary statin prescriptions and repeated lectures about diet.
- **Consider trends.** A single elevated blood pressure reading or cholesterol measurement is less informative than the pattern over time. Track your numbers and pay attention to significant changes, even if they lie within "normal" ranges.
- **Bring context.** When discussing test results with your doctor, share relevant lifestyle factors. Did you fast before the blood draw? Have you been unusually stressed? Have you recently changed medications? This context helps your doctor interpret the numbers accurately.
- **Be selective about screening.** More testing isn't always better. Evidence-based screening recommendations are designed to balance benefits against potential harms such as false positives, unnecessary procedures, and psychological distress.

Your doctor should help you distinguish between statistical abnormalities and actual health concerns. The goal isn't to dismiss all abnormal results but to interpret them intelligently within your individual context.

Medical data, including lab tests, vital signs, and imaging studies, provides invaluable information about your health. But even the most comprehensive testing can tell only part of your story. The best healthcare occurs when scientific evidence meets personal narrative, when your lab values are interpreted alongside your lived experience, when your symptoms are considered as part of the integrated ecosystem that is you. As a patient, you have both the right and the responsibility to participate in this integration. By understanding the value and limitations of medical data, you can work more effectively with your healthcare providers to create a truly personalized approach to your well-being.

But here's what might surprise you: The most important data for understanding your health often isn't found in any lab test or imaging study; it's found in your story, the biographical information that shapes everything from your stress responses to your relationship with food, from your sleep patterns to your approach to medical care. Your test results tell us what's happening in your body right now. Your life story tells us why.

In the next chapter, we'll explore this often overlooked but crucial component of your health data: the biographical information that doctors desperately need but rarely have time to gather and how understanding your own story is a powerful tool for taking charge of your health. The numbers in your chart capture snapshots of your body's current state. But to truly understand your health, we need to examine the experiences, relationships, and circumstances that created those numbers in the first place. Your biographical data, from childhood experiences to current stressors, often holds more predictive power for your future health than any lab test ever could.

5

Your Story: The Biographic Data Doctors Often Overlook

The most-predictive health data often doesn't appear in any test result or medical chart; it lives in your biography. Your childhood experiences, the stress of a pending divorce, your long-term relationship with food, the grief you're processing, or the financial pressures keeping you awake at night all profoundly influence your physical well-being. Yet this biographical information rarely makes it into the medical record, leaving doctors to treat symptoms without understanding their deeper origins.

The invisible dimensions of human experience shape our health in ways that often prove to be more significant than the quantifiable metrics medicine prioritizes. Understanding and integrating your biographical data into your health story is essential for taking charge of your health.

The Missing Pieces of Your Health Puzzle

Your biographical data extends far beyond your basic family history and genetic predispositions. It includes environmental exposures from childhood, significant life events, and ongoing social circumstances that profoundly shape your health. Perhaps you grew up with an alcoholic parent or your grandmother was a Holocaust survivor. Maybe you're caring for aging parents or processing grief. The good news is that modern medicine is finally recognizing the social-emotional determinants of health and the relevance of mental health to physical health. The bad news is that our medical system isn't equipped to integrate this information into your care plan.

To understand the root causes of your headaches, sleeplessness, high blood pressure, or weight struggles, doctors need this much broader set of biographical data. Yet eliciting a patient's story can be challenging for several reasons. It takes time to build trust between patient and doctor. Patients are less likely to disclose important parts of their story if they feel rushed, misunderstood, or judged. To address these problems, medicine has developed questionnaires intended to capture biographical data and social determinants of health. However, patients are even less likely to provide sensitive information to a computer screen than they are to a physician. Let's explore the key categories of biographical data that significantly impact health, but that can remain unseen.

Social-Emotional Health: The Mind-Body Connection

There is no blood test for despair, no CT scan for low self-esteem, no biomarker for grief. A patient mourning the loss of a spouse may present with insomnia, weight loss, and fatigue, symptoms that can be documented in the medical record, but the underlying emotional experience of bereavement remains largely invisible to our measurement tools. The standardized depression questionnaires we use offer crude approximations at best, reducing the rich, multidimensional experience of human suffering to numerical scores that often fail to capture its true nature or significance. My patient Ryan, a software engineer in his mid-sixties, had been labeled as having "health anxiety" in his electronic medical record, a notation that had followed him from doctor to doctor. When he visited a cardiologist for his frequent heart palpitations, the doctor saw the label and reassured him that there was no heart disease. When he saw an endocrinologist for his night sweats, the specialist told him that his hormone levels were normal and suggested relaxation techniques. A neurologist he consulted for his tension headaches dismissed his concerns, attributing them to anxiety and stress.

By the time I saw him for those symptoms, he felt completely unheard. "I know they think I'm crazy," he told me. "But I swear, something is wrong." What no doctor had asked, and what the intake forms had failed to uncover, was his personal history. Ryan had grown up in a household dominated by addiction. His father was an alcoholic with unpredictable mood swings, and his mother had struggled with anxiety. As a child, he had learned to be hypervigilant, scanning for signs of instability and anticipating the next crisis before it happened. That state of constantly being on alert had hardwired his brain to be on edge, a survival mechanism that had served him well in childhood but left him overly sensitive to bodily sensations as an adult. Had any of his doctors asked about his upbringing, they might have recognized that his anxiety about his health wasn't just irrational fear; it was a learned response to living in a household with addiction. What Ryan needed wasn't more testing or repeated reassurance; he needed trauma-informed care and therapy to help retrain his nervous system. Instead of bouncing from specialist to specialist, he could have been directed to someone who could help him process and recalibrate his deeply ingrained fear response.

Public health researchers have developed various patient surveys, such as the GAD-7 (Generalized Anxiety Disorder 7-item scale) for anxiety and the PHQ-9 (Patient Health Questionnaire 9) for depression screening to elicit information about patients' mental health. One problem with these surveys is that people are less likely to accurately answer probing questions such as "Have you felt tired or had little energy?," "Have you had thoughts that you would be better off dead?," and "Have you become easily annoyed or irritable?" when they are asked on a survey, by an administrator behind a medical desk, or by a doctor who barely knows them or, even worse, is asking without first establishing a rapport with them. The other serious limitation of standard mental health questionnaires is that emotional health, regardless of degree, affects every aspect of human health. Patients who don't meet the full diagnostic criteria for generalized anxiety disorder, for example, may still experience the physical manifestations of stress. Patients who don't receive a high enough score on the PHQ-9 may still feel "blue" enough to experience the health harms of untreated trauma or depression.

Anxiety is often considered to be a mental health problem, but it can also be a normal response to a threat. My patient Betty lost her teenage daughter in a car accident forty years ago. To cope, she had become very involved in her church, but she had never sought out formal grief counseling. She didn't think she needed it as long as she had her Sunday routine and her tight group of women friends to support her. Later in life, she was diagnosed with Graves' disease, a metabolic and hormonal problem in which the thyroid gland can become overactive and lead to various symptoms such as chest pain and an irregular heartbeat. When I saw her as a new patient in her seventies, she was taking blood pressure medications and had been instructed by her former physician to monitor her blood pressure readings at home. The problem was that every time she checked her blood pressure, she became very anxious, which drove her blood pressure higher. She had made several trips to the ER for chest pain, and she came in worried about her heart. Her husband insisted that her anxiety was due to age and her Graves' disease.

The immediate concern was that Betty's increase in symptoms often occurred when she was checking her blood pressure. Anxiety tends to cause elevations in blood pressure, and seeing a high blood pressure reading on a home machine can, for many people, trigger anxiety. These are two distinct medical problems that interrelate and can be self-reinforcing. When Betty and I discussed her life story, the data about her past experiences and emotional health, I began to wonder if possibly she had been suffering from unresolved trauma and grief about the death of her daughter. Her anxiety and needing to go to the ER might in part be a manifestation of the ongoing impact of her loss. The death of a child is profound. Symptoms of anxiety, characterized by worry and feelings of vulnerability and uncertainty, are not a necessary or normal feature of aging. However, it is normal for these symptoms to persist if they go unaddressed. Past traumas and painful experiences can have physical manifestations, even decades later.

Betty had edited out a significant part of her life story when discussing her overall health. I suggested she start with grief therapy and a low-dose antidepressant/antianxiety medication. She agreed to try a course of Zoloft with the goal of increasing her emotional "reserves" to reduce the physiological responses to emotional distress and to help her in therapy. I explained that addressing her emotional needs might very likely help with managing her blood pressure issues and her Graves' disease symptoms. "You are more normal than you think," I reassured her.

If you have serious trauma in your past, please try to find a medical provider who wants to listen and who can incorporate addressing that piece of your history into how your present health is being treated. Betty's story illustrates a broader problem in how healthcare professionals approach emotional and physical symptoms. While her blood pressure medications addressed one piece of her health puzzle, the grief that was driving her anxiety—and likely contributing to her blood pressure spikes—remained unaddressed by her medical team.

When Mind and Body Receive Separate Treatment

Despite the fact that mental and physical health are interconnected, our healthcare system continues to treat them as separate domains. You likely have a primary care doctor who manages your blood pressure and cholesterol levels, while any mental health concerns are referred to a different provider, often with different insurance requirements and little communication between the two. This artificial divide creates significant challenges for patients whose symptoms span both domains. Your primary care doctor might prescribe medication for your high blood pressure while remaining unaware that your recent divorce is triggering panic attacks that spike your readings. Meanwhile, your therapist helps you process grief over a job loss but doesn't realize that your resulting sleep disruption is worsening your diabetes control.

The problem isn't just poor communication, it's a fundamental disconnect in how healthcare is organized. Mental health providers often lack training in how emotional states affect physical symptoms, while primary care doctors frequently feel ill equipped to address the psychological factors driving medical conditions. Insurance systems reinforce this split by covering mental and physical health differently, creating additional barriers to integrated care.

How to Advocate for Integrated Care

While you can't single-handedly reform the healthcare system, you can take steps to bridge this divide in your own care:

- **Be explicit about connections.** When discussing physical symptoms with your primary care doctor, mention any relevant stressors, life changes, and emotional concerns. Don't assume that your doctor will ask or make the connection themselves.
- **Share information across providers.** Ensure that you have signed the appropriate medical information releases so your mental health provider and primary care doctor can communicate about your care. Share relevant information with each of them.
- **Look for integration-minded providers.** Some primary care doctors are trained in behavioral health, and some mental health providers understand medical conditions. Seek out providers who recognize these connections.
- **Document patterns yourself.** Keep track of how your emotional state correlates with your physical symptoms. This data can help both of your providers understand the full picture.
- **Consider collaborative care models.** Some healthcare systems offer integrated primary care that includes mental health services in the same location with coordinated treatment plans.

The goal isn't to medicalize normal human emotions or to psychologize legitimate medical concerns; it's to ensure that all aspects of your health are considered when developing treatment plans, rather than treating your mind and body as unrelated systems.

Adverse Childhood Experiences: The Long Shadow of Early Trauma

Adverse childhood experiences (ACEs) are remarkably common, with studies showing that nearly two-thirds of adults have experienced at least one and more than one in five people have endured three or more. These experiences, ranging from emotional neglect and household dysfunction to physical abuse and parental substance use, are strongly linked to long-term health consequences. Research at the CDC and Kaiser Permanente demonstrates that ACEs significantly increase the risk of developing chronic diseases such as heart disease, diabetes, and autoimmune conditions, as well as mental health disorders such as depression, anxiety, and substance use.[1] They also impact behavioral health, contributing to higher rates of smoking, overeating, and risky decision-making.

QUICK REFERENCE
What Are Adverse Childhood Experiences?

- **Types:** Physical, sexual, and emotional abuse; physical and emotional neglect; domestic violence; substance abuse in the household; mental illness in the household; parental separation or divorce; incarcerated household member.
- **Health impacts:** Increased risk of developing heart disease, cancer, diabetes, autoimmune conditions, depression, anxiety, substance use disorders.
- **Why they matter:** Early trauma affects brain development, stress response systems, immune function, and behavioral patterns that persist into adulthood.

1 Vincent J. Felitti, "The Relation Between Adverse Childhood Experiences and Adult Health: *Turning Gold into Lead*," *The Permanente Journal* 6 no. 1 (2002): 44–47, https://pmc.ncbi.nlm.nih.gov/articles/PMC6220625/.

- **Why they're missed:** Shame, stigma, lack of time in medical visits, failure to connect past trauma with current symptoms.

Despite their profound effects, ACEs are notoriously difficult to uncover during a routine doctor's visit. Patients may not recognize the relevance of childhood trauma to their current state of health, may suppress painful memories, or may hesitate to disclose deeply personal experiences in a time-constrained clinical setting. Without a trusting, nonjudgmental space for open discussion, these critical pieces of a patient's health history can remain hidden, leaving doctors to treat symptoms without addressing the underlying causes.

Michael, a fifty-year-old accountant, had struggled with his weight for years. He had tried every diet—low carb, intermittent fasting, calorie counting—but nothing seemed to stick. At his checkup, I noted his rising BMI and borderline high blood sugar level. I asked him about his diet, focusing on what he ate, how often he exercised, and whether he had tried cutting out sugar. Michael explained that he knew what he should be eating—plenty of vegetables, lean proteins, and fewer processed foods—but no matter how hard he tried, he found himself overeating, especially at night. Previous doctors had suggested portion control, a food journal, and possibly a weight loss medication. The last doctor he had seen had handed him a pamphlet on mindful eating and sent him on his way. What those doctors had never asked—and what Michael hadn't volunteered—was why he struggled with overeating in the first place.

It turned out that Michael had grown up in poverty, in a household where food was scarce. As a child, he had never known if there would be enough to eat, and when food was available, he was encouraged to eat as much as possible because the next meal was never guaranteed. That sense of scarcity had stayed with him decades later, despite his having plenty of choices in his fridge and pantry. He wasn't just eating out of hunger; he was eating out of deep-seated fear and ingrained survival instincts. When I understood this important piece of historical data, I asked him about his relationship with food, not just what was on his plate. As he shared more of his story, something clicked. It wasn't about willpower or counting calories; it was about untangling a lifetime of emotional and psychological patterns tied to food.

Michael started working with a therapist who specialized in eating behaviors. He didn't need another restrictive diet; he needed to understand his past, his triggers, and how to reframe his relationship with food. Slowly his habits changed, not because he was forcing himself to eat less but because he no longer felt compelled to overeat. His story is a reminder that not all health data is found in lab results or food logs. The most relevant data wasn't what he was eating but why. A doctor armed with the right questions—not just the right prescription—can make all the difference.

Michael's story demonstrates how food insecurity in childhood can create lasting eating patterns. But childhood doesn't just shape our relationship with food through scarcity; it also profoundly influences how we learn to think about food, our bodies, and eating itself.

How Your Childhood Created Your Relationship with Food

Most of us have a relationship with food that goes beyond hunger and fullness. Our perspectives on eating are shaped during childhood through explicit and implicit messages from our family and culture—lessons about what to eat, when to eat, and how to think about our bodies. These early frameworks often govern our eating behaviors for decades.

According to the National Institutes of Health, obesity rates in the United States have tripled in the last sixty years. Severe obesity has grown tenfold. Globally, women are impacted more than men, even though during this same period, we've cut deaths from heart disease roughly in half. No other health condition has exploded with the ferocity of obesity. Yet for many patients struggling with their weight, the problem isn't lack of knowledge about nutrition; it's their relationship with food itself.

Our connection to food is intertwined with our emotional state. We eat to soothe discomfort, to celebrate, to cope with boredom, loneliness, or stress. Sometimes this relationship lies at the core of patients' health problems, and often it started young. My patient Jessica, a fifty-three-year-old preschool teacher, came to me about fifty pounds overweight and stuck in a familiar cycle: losing and regaining the same thirty pounds repeatedly through extreme dietary measures followed by weight regain and crushing shame. The pattern had created health issues including arthritic knees, high cholesterol, and sleep apnea.

Jessica already ate low carb and exercised regularly, yet doctors kept lecturing her about "calories in, calories out." But obesity isn't a simple math problem; it's a product of biology, psychology, behavior, socioeconomics, and cultural factors. Most of my patients who suffer from being overweight and obesity already know about the harms of extra adipose tissue or the benefits of broccoli, so telling someone like Jessica to "eat better" would be like telling someone with asthma to "breathe better."

When I dug deeper, I learned that her weight struggles traced back to her childhood. Starting in first grade, her mother had called her "chubby" and put her on strict diets. Her father had publicly criticized women's bodies. Through high school, Jessica skipped breakfast and survived on fries, periodically doing extreme "grapefruit diets" to fit into her cheerleading uniform. By college, she was dangerously thin but had to start eating again. Without psychological or nutritional support, she found herself bingeing on sugary foods and gained thirty pounds, triggering deep shame and isolation. It wasn't due to moral failure or lack of willpower; it was due to patterns rooted in her childhood paired with her unmet emotional needs.

Jessica didn't need monthly weight checks in my office; she needed help with emotional eating and practical advice on nourishing her body. With the help of a registered dietician, she learned to eat substantial meals earlier in the day. With more energy, she started incorporating strength training into her routine. Six months later, she had lost fifteen pounds, but more important, her knee pain had improved, her sleep was better, and she no longer felt consumed by thoughts of food and weight. "For the first time," she told me, "I feel like I'm eating to live, not living to eat."

This is what health looks like: not a perfect number on a scale but a sustainable, compassionate relationship with our body and ourselves.

Economic Instability: When Financial Pressures Become Health Problems

Economic instability is one of the most powerful yet frequently overlooked social determinants of health. Research consistently demonstrates that high income, wealth, and economic security or the lack thereof profoundly impact health outcomes across the lifespan. According to the American Public Health Association, individuals living in poverty are approximately three times more likely to die prematurely than those with higher incomes.[2] This disparity reflects more than just limited access to healthcare; it encompasses inadequate housing, food insecurity, transportation barriers, chronic stress, and a reduced ability to engage in health-promoting behaviors.

Despite overwhelming evidence of these connections, our healthcare system continues to operate as if health exists in an economic vacuum. Medical schools provide minimal training on recognizing and addressing financial barriers to care. Electronic health records rarely capture economic determinants in meaningful ways. And reimbursement structures ignore social and economic roots. The result is a healthcare system that often prescribes inaccessible solutions. Physicians recommend medications without considering whether patients can afford them, suggest dietary changes without accounting for food deserts, and create treatment plans requiring transportation resources that many patients lack. This disconnect doesn't just create inefficiency; it actively compounds the suffering of our most vulnerable populations.

---

2 Anton L. V. Avanceña et al., "Income and Income Inequality Are a Matter of Life and Death. What Can Policymakers Do About It?" *American Journal of Public Health* 111 (August 31, 2021): 1404–1408, https://ajph.aphapublications.org/doi/full/10.2105/AJPH.2021.306301.

Gordon, a retired government worker with thinning white hair and careful posture, was seventy-nine when he became my patient. His medical chart was notable for congestive heart failure, type 2 diabetes, chronic kidney disease, osteoarthritis, and COPD. More complex was his medication list: seventeen prescriptions from five different specialists, many at maximum doses. Despite that intensive medical management, Gordon's health was deteriorating. His blood pressure was poorly controlled. His glucose readings swung wildly. His breathing had worsened. Each specialist responded by adjusting his medications or adding new ones, creating a cascade of prescriptions that seemed to compound rather than resolve his symptoms.

When Gordon first came to my office, I began with standard medical questions, but something in his demeanor—perhaps the way he carefully folded and refolded his medication list—prompted me to ask about the logistics of his daily life.

"How do you manage all these medications, Gordon? That's quite a list to keep track of."

He looked down at his hands. "Honestly, Doc, I don't always get them filled on time."

That opened a conversation revealing the economic reality behind Gordon's medical struggles. His modest pension and Social Security benefits barely covered his mortgage and utilities. After paying for groceries, he often had to choose which prescriptions to fill based on which symptoms bothered him most that month. Additionally, he lived in a neighborhood poorly served by public transportation. Without a car, he relied on a community shuttle that ran to the pharmacy only twice weekly. If he missed the shuttle, he'd go days or weeks without essential medications.

What appeared medically as nonadherence was economic survival. No one had asked Gordon these fundamental questions: Can you afford these medications? How do you physically get to the pharmacy? What happens when medication costs compete with your other basic needs?

Understanding these realities required rethinking Gordon's entire care plan. Together, we worked to simplify his medication regimen, prioritizing combination pills to reduce costs and dosing schedules that aligned with his transportation access. I connected him with Medicare's Extra Help program and pharmaceutical company assistance programs. For his diabetes, we switched to more affordable options that didn't require refrigeration or frequent monitoring of supplies. I arranged for medication delivery services and helped him enroll in a program providing transportation to medical appointments.

Within months, Gordon's blood pressure stabilized. His glucose control improved. His symptoms eased, because we'd addressed the economic barriers preventing him from taking the treatments already prescribed. His story reveals how economic factors become encoded as medical problems. His chart listed "medication nonadherence" as if it were a character flaw rather than due to economic necessity.

What Gordon needed were practical solutions addressing the realities of his daily life. For him and so many others, economic circumstances are not peripheral factors; they are central determinants that shape every aspect of health and healing.

Social Isolation and Loneliness: The Health Impact of Disconnection

Social isolation and loneliness have emerged as significant public health concerns with profound impacts on physical and mental well-being. Research has consistently demonstrated that social connection is not merely a psychological comfort but a fundamental biological need. According to a meta-analysis published in *PLOS Medicine*, social isolation increases mortality risk by 29 percent, comparable to the risk associated with smoking fifteen cigarettes daily.[3] The American Heart Association has recognized social isolation as a risk factor for coronary heart disease and stroke, while

3 Ryo Naito et al., "Social Isolation as a Risk Factor for All-Cause Mortality: Systematic Review and Meta-Analysis of Cohort Studies," *PLoS ONE* 18 vol. 1 (January 12, 2023), https://journals.plos.org/plosone/article?id=10.1371/journal.pone.0280308.

studies show that chronic loneliness triggers inflammatory responses and immune system dysregulation that accelerate disease progression.[4]

Keith's story illustrates how social disconnection becomes encoded in the body as measurable medical problems. A forty-five-year-old engineer, he had been married for fifteen years when his wife asked for a divorce. The split had been amicable, no infidelity and no dramatic fights, but that had somehow made it harder. "We grew apart," he explained when he came to my office six months later. What brought Keith to see me wasn't the divorce itself but a constellation of physical symptoms that had developed since then. His blood pressure, which had been normal for years, was now consistently elevated at 165/95 mmHg. He'd gained twenty-five pounds despite eating less than he had during his marriage. Most concerning to him were the chest pains that had sent him to the emergency room twice, only for him to be prescribed blood pressure pills and told by various doctors that his heart was fine.

While that advice wasn't wrong, it missed the deeper story. Since his divorce, Keith's social structure had vanished. His wife had been his primary companion, and most of their friends were couples who no longer included him in their social activities. His teenage kids lived with him every other week, but during his off weeks, he often went days without meaningful conversations with another person. The isolation was taking a measurable toll on his body. His sleep became fitful as he lay awake worrying. Without adequate rest, his stress hormones spiked, driving up his blood pressure and depositing weight around his middle. The chest pains weren't due to heart disease; they were the physical manifestations of anxiety and panic. It made sense. Keith had stopped cooking, relying instead on takeout and frozen meals that he ate alone in front of the television. Exercise, which he'd enjoyed doing with his wife, felt pointless and lonely. Even grocery shopping became a reminder of his solitary state: buying

---

4 "Social Isolation, Loneliness Can Damage Heart and Brain Health, Report Says," American Heart Association, updated August 4, 2022, https://www.heart.org/en/news/2022/08/04/social-isolation-loneliness-can-damage-heart-and-brain-health-report-says.

single servings of everything, seeing families together, feeling like an outsider looking in.

Working with Keith required addressing both his physical symptoms and their social roots. Yes, he needed blood pressure medication temporarily, but more important, he needed human connection. We talked about his joining a divorce support group and reconnecting with old friends. I referred him to a therapist to help him process the grief of his divorce while developing a social network.

Gradually, Keith's health markers began to improve. Getting out of his head and into the company of people who cared about him was therapeutic. Rekindling old friendships felt good; it also gradually improved his sleep. His blood pressure decreased to the point where we could reduce his medication dose. The chest pains disappeared as his anxiety lessened. Most tellingly, he began cooking again, not just for himself but for friends he invited over for dinner. His story demonstrates how social connection is a vital health determinant that directly impacts measurable medical outcomes. What had appeared as straightforward hypertension was the toll of social isolation in disguise. The most effective treatment was the psychological safety that no pill could provide.

Invisible Data, Invisible Suffering: What Standard Care Misses

The everyday emotional experiences fundamental to human existence—anxiety about an uncertain future, sadness over paths not taken, worry about loved ones, frustration with physical limitations—rarely merit medical attention unless they cross arbitrary thresholds of severity or duration. Yet these "subclinical" emotional states profoundly influence health behaviors, treatment adherence, and physiological processes from inflammation to immune function.

Consider a menopausal woman experiencing mood swings, brain fog, and sleep disruption. Her laboratory values may be within normal limits and her physical examination unremarkable. Because these symptoms don't neatly correspond to measurable biomarkers, they're often dismissed or minimized by a healthcare system that prizes quantifiable data above subjective experience. Or take the elderly man who lost his sense of purpose after retirement. His vital signs remained stable, his routine bloodwork unremarkable. Yet the absence of meaning in his daily life created profound suffering that ultimately manifested itself as physical decline, not because of any measurable disease process but because human beings require more than physiological maintenance to thrive.

This invisible suffering occurs in patients navigating chronic pain, where the subjective experience often bears little relationship to imaging findings or other objective measures. It causes the distress of patients with medically unexplained symptoms, who often face skepticism or outright dismissal when their suffering cannot be validated by our existing measurement tools. It includes the existential distress of terminal illness, in which quality-of-life considerations may be sacrificed in pursuit of marginally improved survival metrics. The toll of invisible suffering is particularly acute for marginalized populations, whose experiences may not conform to standardized assessment tools. Cultural variations in the expression of emotional distress, when filtered through standardized screening instruments, may register as either over- or under-pathologized, leading to inappropriate treatment decisions.

Reclaiming Your Narrative: How to Integrate Your Story into Your Care

As we've explored throughout these three chapters, your health data encompasses far more than what typically appears in your medical chart. The INFORMATICS quadrant of your health ecosystem includes:

- **Medical measurements:** The quantifiable metrics that doctors track, from cholesterol levels to genetic markers, which provide essential but incomplete information about your physical state

- **Clinical context:** The interpretation of these numbers within the framework of medical evidence, your personal risk factors, and your unique circumstances
- **Biographical data:** The often invisible aspects of your life story, from your childhood experiences to your current stressors, that profoundly shape how your body functions

Understanding the interplay among these different types of data empowers you to become a better-informed participant in your healthcare. It enables you to see beyond isolated test results to the complete picture of the factors influencing your well-being. It puts you into the driver's seat of understanding your medical data and with a greater ability to become the CEO of your own health. As you reflect on your INFORMATICS quadrant, consider not just what your numbers say but what story they tell when combined with your life experiences, stressors, and personal history. These connections form the groundwork for understanding how the other quadrants of your health ecosystem operate.

While medical professionals may not ask you enough about yourself or might miss important parts of your medical data, you can look at your life and your past yourself. You can do a self-inventory that will bring a fuller understanding of your biographical data into focus. And from there, you can start asking where this data fits into your overall health status.

Some ways to integrate your story into your healthcare include:

- **Prepare for appointments** by jotting down notes about how your symptoms connect to other aspects of your life: stress, relationships, work, and past experiences.
- **Be direct with your doctor** about relevant biographical information, even if they don't specifically ask.
- **Consider how your upbringing and past experiences** might be influencing your current health behaviors and physical symptoms.

- **Look for patterns** between emotional states and physical symptoms.
- **Seek out providers** who demonstrate interest in your whole story, not just your symptoms.

Remember, you are the expert on your own lived experience. While medical providers have expertise in disease processes and treatments, you possess irreplaceable knowledge about how illness and wellness manifest themselves in the unique context of your life.

Finding a Good Primary Care Provider

Painting your complete INFORMATICS picture—both your biometric data and your biographical story—is most powerful when you have a primary care provider who knows you. Even with perfect self-knowledge, you still need professional guidance. Even as AI becomes more sophisticated at pattern recognition and data analysis, you need a human advocate.

Finding the right primary care provider requires time and intention. When evaluating potential candidates, look beyond their credentials to find someone who listens without interrupting, explains things clearly in language you understand, and respects your questions and concerns. Pay attention to whether they explain the reasoning behind their recommendations and seem willing to collaborate with other providers when needed. Most important, trust your instincts about whether you feel comfortable being honest with them.

The best clinicians demonstrate humility alongside their expertise. They tell you what they know and what they don't know. They're also willing to revise their views as science evolves. Be wary of any doctor who claims absolute certainty, especially about complex topics, or who seems threatened by new data or other experts' opinions. Medicine is a team sport!

Your primary care provider should also be able to manage many conditions in-house before referring you to specialists. In theory, specialists exist to help diagnose and treat problems beyond a primary care physician's expertise or when specialized testing is needed. In practice, our healthcare system's shortage of primary care doctors means that specialists increasingly handle work that could be done by generalists (which is why it takes so long to get specialist appointments these days).

You shouldn't need a cardiologist to manage your blood pressure, an orthopedist for your back pain, or an endocrinologist for your diabetes care. These conditions are often best managed by someone who understands how they interconnect with the rest of your health. When your diabetes medication causes dizziness or your pain medication raises your blood pressure, you need a doctor who can see these connections and not reflexively send you back to a specialist.

Finally, trust your gut. If something doesn't feel right, it may not be the right fit. At the same time, recognize that doctors are human, too. We have bad days and busy lives just like everyone else. Acknowledging your doctor's humanity can go a long way toward building a sturdy relationship.

Finding Primary Care When Options Are Limited

- **Community health centers:** Federally qualified health centers (FQHCs) provide comprehensive primary care regardless of your ability to pay. Find locations at findahealthcenter.hrsa.gov.
- **Direct primary care (DPC):** This membership-based model eliminates insurance billing, allowing for longer appointments (typically thirty to sixty minutes), better access through email/phone/telehealth, and more personalized care. Search for "DPC practices" at dpcalliance.org. While typically requiring out-of-pocket payment ($50 to $150 per month), DPC often provides the relationship-centered care that makes implementing this framework much easier.
- **Nurse practitioners and physician assistants:** I am a big fan of NPs and PAs. These providers often have more appointment availability, spend more time with patients, and can be excellent partners in comprehensive health management. Many specialize in primary care and can provide the same services physicians do.

- **Telehealth primary care:** Platforms such as PlushCare, MDLive, and One Medical offer virtual primary care relationships that can provide continuity and comprehensive care coordination.

What to Look For

When evaluating potential primary care providers, prioritize these qualities:

- Listens without interrupting and asks follow-up questions about your life circumstances.
- Explains medical information clearly and welcomes your questions.
- Demonstrates interest in your complete story, not just your symptoms.
- Shows a willingness to collaborate with other providers and specialists.
- Respects your time and maintains reasonable appointment availability.

Practical Steps

1. **Check your insurance network** to understand your covered options and potential costs.
2. **Gather recommendations** from friends with similar health needs, other healthcare providers you trust, or local community groups.
3. **Schedule a "meet and greet" appointment** with potential providers to assess fit.
4. **Prepare for initial visits** by documenting your health history, current concerns, and questions about their practice style.
5. **Trust your instincts** about the relationship; you should feel comfortable being honest and asking questions.

Maximizing Any Healthcare Relationship

Even without an established primary care doctor, you can still implement this framework effectively:

- **Document your complete health story** using the reflection and action guides throughout this book.
- **Prepare focused, specific questions** for any healthcare encounters.
- **Bring your four-quadrant analysis** to urgent care, specialist visits, and telehealth consultations.

- **Keep your own comprehensive health record** that travels with you between providers.

Remember: Your health ecosystem doesn't disappear if you don't have a regular doctor; it just requires you to take more responsibility for coordinating its various elements. The framework you're learning will give you the tools to be an effective advocate regardless of your current access to healthcare.

KNOW YOURSELF, ADVOCATE FOR YOURSELF

Your INFORMATICS Reflection and Action Guide

PART 1 Self-Reflection: Understanding Your INFORMATICS Quadrant

It's time to retrieve your pen and paper or laptop. Here we will flesh out the first quadrant of your health ecosystem. Start by writing down the answers to the following questions:

Biometric Data: The Measurable Stuff

- What health data do you currently track or have access to (lab results, imaging test results, vital signs, wearable device metrics, genetic information)?
- Which of these numbers do you understand well? Which confuse you or create anxiety?
- Have you ever received a "normal" test result that didn't match how you actually felt? What was that experience like?
- What health data or symptoms have you tracked on your own that you've never shared with a doctor? Why haven't you shared this information?

Biographic Data: Your Life as Context

- What major life experiences (childhood events, traumas, significant relationships, losses) do you think might be affecting your current health?
- How has stress shown up physically in your body throughout your life? What patterns have you noticed?
- What aspects of your biography (work environment, financial pressures, caregiving responsibilities, relationship dynamics) might your healthcare providers not fully understand?
- When you look at your health metrics or symptoms, what connections do you see to your life circumstances that doctors might miss?

Information Sources and Trust

- Where do you get your health information? How do you evaluate whether sources are trustworthy?

- Have you ever felt dismissed or not believed when sharing medical data, your symptoms, or your story with a healthcare provider? How did that affect your care?
- What questions have you been afraid to ask your doctor? What holds you back?

Integration and Gaps

- What feels missing from your medical records that would help providers understand you better?
- If you could tell your doctor one thing about your life story that would change how they interpret your health data, what would it be?
- Are there screenings or tests you think you might need but haven't pursued? What's preventing you from getting them?

PART 2 Healthcare Conversations: Questions and Strategies for Medical Encounters

Questions to Ask Your Medical Provider

- "Could you help me understand what this test result means in the context of my health situation and risk factors?"
- "How might my [specific life circumstance] be affecting these results?"
- "How significant is the change in my numbers from last time?"
- "How urgent is it that I implement the [lifestyle/medication/habit] changes you recommend in order to improve these numbers?"
- "Which intervention is the most important for me to start right away, and what data do we expect will change?"
- "What are some good sources for evidence-based medical information?"
- "How should I know if a panic headline or abnormal lab test is worth worrying about?"
- "How will we measure my health progress? With lab tests or other metrics?"
- "What is one small, specific action I could take this [week/month/year] to start taking charge of my health?"

Communication Strategies

- Tell your medical provider that you understand that context matters when interpreting data and that you welcome a robust conversation about test results.
- Explain that your goal is to learn more about your health from your provider, to partner with them to get educated about your data, and to feel empowered to make healthy decisions.
- Bring a timeline and description of your symptoms plus a timeline and description of major life events that may relate to your health.
- Request copies of all test results and written summaries of complex medical information.
- When receiving a new diagnosis, make sure you ask for fact-based information and resources to learn more about the condition.

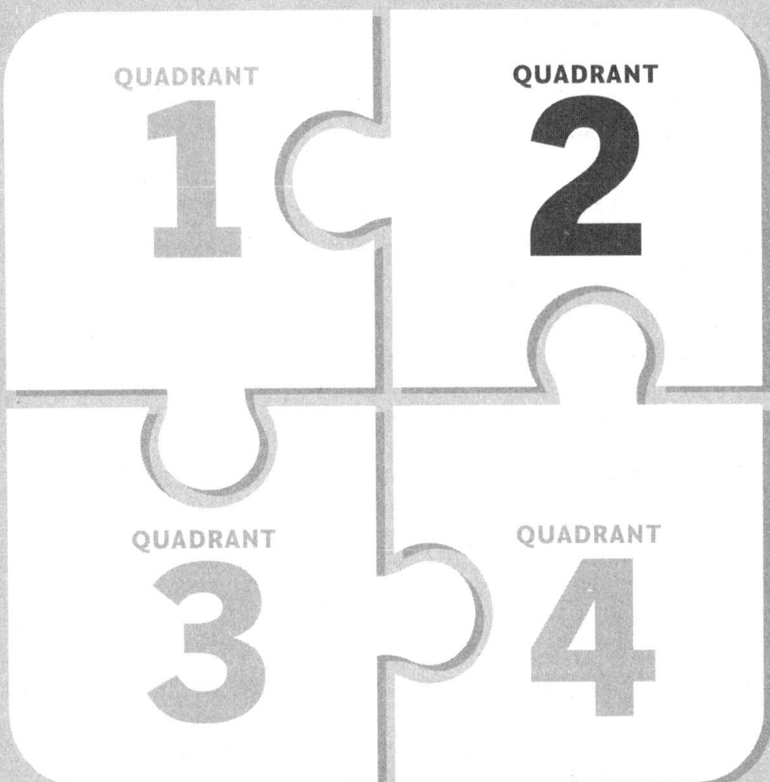

INPUTS

You are what you eat. You're also what you drink, smoke, swallow, and absorb—aka INPUTS. This quadrant encompasses every substance that enters your body from the morning caffè latte that jump-starts your day to the prescription medication that manages your blood pressure, from the late-night stress eating that follows a tough conversation to the supplements you're hoping will whittle your waistline.

This quadrant reveals itself most directly in your lab results. Your cholesterol levels reflect not just your genetics but also your relationship with food when you are under stress. Your blood sugar patterns tell the story of skipped meals, emotional eating, and the intersection of your life circumstances with your nutritional choices. Your liver enzymes might spike not due to disease but due to that new supplement regimen you started after watching a wellness influencer's latest video.

Yet INPUTS go far deeper than what shows up on blood tests. Every substance you consume carries meaning beyond its molecular structure. Food isn't just fuel; it's comfort, celebration, rebellion, control, or chaos. Alcohol isn't just ethanol; it's social connection, stress relief, or self-medication. Supplements aren't just vitamins; they're hope and the promise of health optimization.

Understanding your INPUTS means recognizing both the biochemical and the emotional relationships you have with everything you consume. It means understanding how your childhood experiences influence what you eat, drink, and consume today. It means reckoning with Big Wellness's outsized influence on your diet and supplements list. It means understanding the rationale for every prescription drug you take. Most important, it means connecting the dots between your INPUTS and your other health quadrants.

By the end of this section, you'll understand how to make informed decisions about what you consume—decisions based on evidence rather than marketing, on your real needs rather than aspirational lifestyle content, and on creating sustainable relationships with everything you put in your body.

You Really Are What You Eat

Here's a confession that medical practitioners don't want you to know: Doctors of my generation received virtually no training in nutrition during medical school. Despite spending years memorizing the Krebs cycle and rare genetic disorders, most of us graduated without the practical knowledge to guide patients through their actual daily food choices. The average physician receives less than twenty hours of nutrition education during four years of medical school. Instead of learning how different foods affect different bodies and how to tailor dietary advice to individual patients, we were taught to diagnose and prescribe. This education gap doesn't just shortchange patients; it fundamentally shapes how the US medical system approaches food.

Yet food is medicine. In my practice, consuming soluble fiber helped one patient's constipation more than laxatives or expensive probiotics did. Consuming more dietary calcium improved another patient's bone density scores more than Fosamax could have. Consuming healthy fats helped a third patient's restrictive eating habits more than Prozac did. Food is more than merely fuel; it can prevent and even cure disease. But medical providers consistently fall short in this realm. We excel at telling patients to "eat healthy," yet we fail to explain how specific foods directly impact their lab values, symptoms, and long-term health outcomes. We need to help our patients understand that what they put into their bodies shapes every other aspect of their health ecosystem.

What Is "Healthy Eating"? Basic Tenets for Whole Person Health

The foundation of good nutritional health rests on a few fundamental pillars that go beyond trendy diets or quick fixes. Proper nourishment is about providing the basic building blocks for every organ system, from brain function to bone health. These blocks, or "macronutrients," work synergistically and play distinct, essential roles in fueling the body and mind. Let's review each one and why they matter.

Protein: The Essential Builder

Protein is critical for virtually every function in the body. While its role in muscle health receives the most attention, its benefits extend throughout the body. Adequate protein intake supports bone health; immune function; hair, skin, and nail integrity; weight management; and blood sugar regulation.

Consider Janet, a fifty-eight-year-old teacher going through menopause. She came to me concerned about her bone density scan showing osteopenia, the precursor of osteoporosis. Her estrogen levels had dropped significantly, and she assumed that calcium supplements would solve her bone health problems. But when I examined her dietary intake, I found that she was consuming barely 40 grams of protein daily, far below what her changing body needed. She was stunned to learn that her "healthy" eating pattern was contributing to her bone loss. She'd been focusing on eating salads and vegetables, avoiding red meat due to concerns about cholesterol, but no one had ever explained to her that protein consumption was crucial for good bone health. She had always assumed it was just about calcium and vitamin D.

As estrogen declines during menopause, women need more protein to maintain their muscle mass and bone density. In this case, the connection between INPUTS and INFORMATICS became clear: Janet's low protein intake wasn't just affecting her muscle tissue, it was directly impacting her bone mineral density measurements. We worked together to increase her protein intake to 80 to 90 grams daily, spread throughout the day. Within six months, along with resistance training, her follow-up DEXA scan showed improved bone density.

Janet's case illustrates how our food can be medical fuel. She reported feeling stronger overall, not just in her bones, and interestingly, she noticed that she was less preoccupied with thoughts of food throughout the day. When she'd been eating mostly salads, she was constantly hungry and thinking about her next meal.

From a medical data perspective, protein offers benefits that often surprise patients. Most adults need 0.7 to 1.0 gram of protein per kilogram (2.2 pounds) of body weight daily. For someone weighing 160 pounds (73 kilograms), this translates to 50 to 73 grams of protein daily. After age forty, we need more (closer to 1.2 grams per kilogram) to counter age-related muscle loss.

QUICK REFERENCE
Protein Sources and Content (from highest to lowest protein content)

- **3 ounces fatty fish (salmon, tuna, sardines):** 20–25 grams
- **3 ounces chicken breast:** 21 grams
- **1 cup Greek yogurt:** 20 grams
- **1 cup lentils (cooked):** 18 grams
- **3.5 ounces firm tofu:** 15 grams
- **1 cup edamame (shelled):** 12 grams
- **1 cup quinoa:** 8 grams
- **2 tablespoons peanut butter:** 8 grams
- **1 ounce almonds (about 23 nuts):** 6 grams
- **1 ounce walnuts (about 14 halves):** 4 grams

Pro tip: Most adults need 0.7 to 1.0 gram of protein per kilogram (2.2 pounds) of body weight daily, more after age forty. For optimal muscle health, aim to distribute your protein intake evenly across your meals—about 25 to 30 grams per meal.

The timing matters, too. Research suggests that spreading protein intake evenly across meals optimizes muscle maintenance and growth. This distribution affects not just muscle health but also blood sugar regulation and cognitive function, showing how INPUTS directly influence multiple aspects of your health ecosystem.

There are many ways to increase your protein intake. Start with breakfast, the meal most likely to be protein deficient. Adding eggs, Greek yogurt, or a high-quality protein powder to your morning routine can transform your entire day's energy pattern. Keep convenient protein sources, such as hard-boiled eggs, individual Greek yogurt containers, edamame, or preportioned nuts, on hand for snacks.

If your diet is plant based, be intentional about combining protein sources and slightly increasing your overall target to account for plant-based proteins' lower digestibility. For those struggling to meet their protein needs through food alone, consider consuming high-quality protein supplements such as whey, pea, hemp, or blended plant proteins as a practical bridge. Remember that adequate protein works synergistically with resistance exercise, creating a virtuous cycle in which protein feeds muscle growth, which increases metabolic rate, which makes weight management easier, which further supports overall health.

Building on this protein foundation, your body also requires another building block: fiber. This dietary element is one that people often overlook but is crucial for a healthy body and mind.

Fiber: The Unsung Hero

Fiber might be the most underrated nutritional component. It doesn't just prevent constipation; it feeds the beneficial bacteria in our gut, helps regulate blood sugar, and creates a feeling of fullness that prevents overeating. More important, it works in concert with the protein just discussed, slowing digestion and helping us maintain steady energy levels throughout the day.

My patient Marcus, a forty-two-year-old tech executive, came to me with a list of complaints: constant hunger despite adequate calorie intake, afternoon energy crashes, irritable bowel symptoms, and difficulty managing his weight despite regular exercise. He explained that he was eating what most people would consider "healthy": egg whites in the morning, a turkey sandwich at lunch, chicken and broccoli for dinner. Yet he was starving all the time, and his digestive system was a mess.

Looking at his diary, I noticed something striking: His fiber intake averaged just 11 grams daily, less than half the recommended amount. His high-protein diet, while technically "clean" by fitness standards, lacked the fiber his body desperately needed. When I suggested focusing on fiber-rich foods, Marcus was skeptical. He thought fiber was just about digestive regularity, not realizing its broader impact on the gut microbiome, energy regulation, and satiety.

We developed a plan for him to gradually increase His fiber intake through whole foods by adding berries to his breakfast, switching to whole grain bread for his sandwiches, incorporating beans and lentils into his meals, and snacking on nuts and seeds instead of protein bars. I warned him to increase slowly and drink more water to prevent digestive discomfort during the transition. Three weeks later, he reported remarkable changes. He felt full after meals, his energy remained steady throughout the day, and his digestive issues had almost completely resolved. Even his cravings for sweets had diminished. His experience reflects the profound systemic effects of this often-overlooked nutrient.

I suggest consuming 25 to 30 grams per day, through diet and supplementation as needed. Most Americans consume only 12 grams daily, less than half the recommended amount! Those who consistently consume 25 grams or more per day experience better health outcomes and less visceral fat accumulation.

There are two primary types of fiber, each with unique benefits. **Soluble fiber** dissolves in water to form a gel-like substance that slows digestion and helps lower glucose and blood cholesterol levels. **Insoluble fiber** adds bulk to stool and helps food pass more quickly through the stomach and intestines. The two types of fiber work synergistically in the body, which is why a diverse diet rich in plant foods naturally provides the optimal mix.

When choosing supplements, look for products that contain both soluble and insoluble fiber rather than focusing exclusively on one type.

QUICK REFERENCE
Fiber Sources and Content
(from highest to lowest fiber content)

Legumes and Seeds

- **1 cup cooked black beans:** 15 grams (mixed: high soluble)
- **1 cup cooked lentils:** 15 grams (mixed: high soluble)
- **1 cup cooked chickpeas:** 12 grams (mixed: high soluble)
- **1 cup edamame (shelled):** 10 grams (mixed)
- **2 tablespoons chia seeds:** 10 grams (mixed: high soluble)
- **2 tablespoons ground flaxseeds:** 4 grams (mixed)

Fruits

- **1 medium avocado:** 10 grams (mixed)
- **1 cup raspberries:** 8 grams (mixed: high insoluble)
- **1 cup blackberries:** 8 grams (mixed: high insoluble)
- **1 medium pear with skin:** 6 grams (mixed)
- **1 medium apple with skin:** 5 grams (mixed: high soluble)
- **1 medium banana:** 3 grams (mixed)

Vegetables

- **1 cup cooked artichoke hearts:** 10 grams (mixed)
- **1 cup cooked broccoli:** 5 grams (mixed: high insoluble)
- **1 cup cooked Brussels sprouts:** 4 grams (mixed: high insoluble)
- **1 medium sweet potato with skin:** 4 grams (mixed)
- **1 cup cooked green beans:** 4 grams (mixed: high insoluble)
- **1 cup cooked cauliflower:** 3 grams (mixed: high insoluble)

Whole Grains and Nuts

- **1 cup whole grain pasta:** 6 grams (mixed: high insoluble)
- **1 cup cooked quinoa:** 5 grams (mixed)

- **1 cup cooked brown rice:** 4 grams (mixed: high insoluble)
- **1 cup cooked oatmeal:** 4 grams (mixed: high soluble)
- **1 ounce almonds (23 nuts):** 4 grams (mixed: high insoluble)
- **1 slice whole grain bread:** 3–4 grams (mixed: high insoluble)

Increasing your fiber intake too quickly can cause digestive distress. Instead, gradually add 5 grams of fiber every week until you reach your target. Simultaneously, increase your water intake. Fiber works best when it can absorb water, and staying well hydrated prevents the constipation that might otherwise occur with higher fiber consumption.

In addition to classic fiber-rich foods such as vegetables, fruits, legumes, and whole grains, look for easy fiber boosters to add to foods you already enjoy: Sprinkle ground flaxseeds or chia seeds onto yogurt or into smoothies, add beans to soups and salads, choose whole fruits rather than juices, swap white rice for brown or wild rice, and incorporate more leafy greens and cruciferous vegetables into your meals. Even small changes, such as leaving the skin on potatoes or choosing whole grain pasta over refined, can significantly increase your fiber intake over time.

Remember that food processing often removes fiber, so the closer a food is to its natural state, the more fiber it typically contains. Reading nutrition labels can help you identify high-fiber options when shopping for packaged foods; look for at least 3 grams of fiber per serving as a good starting point.

While fiber provides the structural foundation for healthy digestion and steady energy, there's another macronutrient that's been unfairly maligned despite being essential for virtually every cellular function in the human body.

Healthy Fats: Essential for Brain and Hormone Health

The demonization of fat has been one of nutrition science's greatest missteps. Our brains are approximately 60 percent fat, and every cell membrane in our body requires fat to function properly. Fats are also necessary for hormone production, nutrient absorption, and cellular health. Consuming the right fats in appropriate amounts is one of the most powerful dietary shifts you can make for long-term health.

Talia, a thirty-five-year-old graphic designer, came to see me for persistent brain fog, irregular menstrual cycles, dry skin, and depression symptoms that hadn't responded to medication. Her previous doctor had put her on a very-low-fat diet to address her slightly elevated cholesterol. She was doing everything "right" by conventional wisdom, using fat-free everything and avoiding oils almost entirely. But she felt worse than ever, and her therapist had suggested that she might have ADHD because her concentration was so poor.

When I reviewed her food journal, I was struck by the nearly complete absence of fats, particularly omega-3 fatty acids. Her diet consisted primarily of fat-free products, lean protein, and carbohydrates. The unintended consequence? Her hormone production was impaired, her cell membranes were struggling, and her brain, which requires fat to function properly, was starving. Talia was confused by the conflicting messages she'd received about fat. I explained that fat isn't a villain but an essential nutrient her body cannot function without. The type and quality of fat matter far more than the quantity.

We redesigned her diet to include healthy fats from avocados, olive oil, nuts, seeds, and fatty fish. I explained that these foods provide essential fatty acids her body cannot produce itself, supporting brain function, hormone production, and cell membrane integrity. Within three months, Talia reported remarkable improvements. Her brain fog had lifted, her concentration had returned, her skin had regained its luster, and her menstrual cycles had normalized. Most surprisingly to her, her cholesterol profile actually improved, with increased HDL ("good" cholesterol) and decreased triglycerides. She felt as though someone had turned the lights back on in her brain after years of avoiding the very thing her body needed.

According to current nutritional guidelines, healthy adults should get about 20 to 35 percent of their daily calories from fats. For someone consuming 2,000 calories per day, this translates to approximately 44 to 78 grams of total fat. For essential omega-3 fatty acids (a type of polyunsaturated fat), the adequate intake for adults is approximately:

- 1.6 grams daily for men
- 1.1 grams daily for women

QUICK REFERENCE

Fat Types

- **Monounsaturated fats,** which support heart health (olive oil, avocados, nuts)
- **Omega-3 fatty acids,** which reduce inflammation and support brain health (fatty fish, walnuts, flax)
- **Saturated fats** in moderation from whole foods (coconut oil, dairy products)

Healthy Fat Sources and Content (from highest to lowest fat content)

- **1 medium avocado:** 21 grams (monounsaturated)
- **1 ounce walnuts (14 halves):** 18 grams (omega-3)
- **2 tablespoons almond butter:** 16 grams (monounsaturated)
- **3 ounces salmon:** 15 grams (omega-3)
- **1 tablespoon olive oil:** 14 grams (monounsaturated)
- **1 ounce almonds (23 nuts):** 14 grams (monounsaturated)
- **1 ounce sunflower seeds:** 14 grams (monounsaturated)
- **1 ounce cashews (18 nuts):** 12 grams (monounsaturated)
- **2 tablespoons chia seeds:** 9 grams (omega-3)
- **1 ounce dark chocolate (70%+ cacao):** 9 grams (monounsaturated)
- **2 tablespoons ground flaxseeds:** 4 grams (omega-3)
- **1 large egg:** 5 grams (mixed)
- **3 ounces tuna:** 5 grams (omega-3)

Target: 20 to 35 percent of daily calories from healthy fats (44 to 78 grams for 2,000 calories). Essential omega-3s: 1.1 grams daily for women, 1.6 grams for men. Focus on whole food sources over isolated oils when possible.

Healthy fats from sources such as olive oil, avocados, nuts, seeds, and fatty fish provide essential fatty acids our bodies cannot produce themselves. These fats help reduce inflammation, support hormone production, and enable the absorption of fat-soluble vitamins (A, D, E, and K). Many of my patients who struggle with mood disorders, inflammatory conditions, or hormonal imbalances see improvement when they increase their intake of these beneficial fats.

How to Incorporate Healthy Fats into Your Diet

- **Start your day with healthy fats.** Add avocado to your toast, nut butter to your oatmeal, or ground flaxseeds to your smoothie.
- **Make simple swaps.** Replace processed dressings with olive oil and vinegar, margarine with avocado or olive oil, and processed snacks with nuts.
- **Focus on whole food sources.** Whenever possible, get your fats from whole foods rather than isolated oils.
- **Balance your fats.** Include sources of all types of healthy fats throughout the week, with special attention to increasing your omega-3 intake if you typically eat a Western diet.
- **Consider your overall diet.** Remember that healthy fats work synergistically with fiber, protein, and phytonutrients (nutrients found in plant compounds and nuts and parts of the bean family); they're just one piece of the nutritional puzzle.

Remember that fat is the most calorie-dense macronutrient at 9 calories per gram, compared to 4 calories per gram for both protein and carbohydrates. While healthy fats are essential, portion awareness remains important for overall caloric balance.

Healthy fats work particularly well when paired with complex carbohydrates, which brings us to one of the most misunderstood food categories in modern nutrition.

Whole Grains: Essential for Sustained Energy and Nutritional Complexity

Let's be crystal clear about something that confuses many people: Carbohydrates are not the enemy; ultraprocessed carbohydrates are. There's a world of difference between a bowl of steel-cut oats and a frosted pastry, between quinoa and white bread, between a sweet potato and potato chips. When we talk about carbohydrates, we're actually talking about a spectrum that ranges from whole food sources packed with nutrients to highly processed products stripped of their natural benefits.

The critical distinction is this: Whole food carbohydrates come packaged by nature with fiber, protein, vitamins, minerals, and antioxidants that work together to provide sustained energy and support your health. Processed carbohydrates have been stripped of these beneficial components, leaving behind concentrated starches and sugars that spike your blood sugar level and leave you hungry again quickly.

News flash: Not all grains are created equal, and the differences matter enormously for your health. Here's what you need to know:

- **Whole grains** contain the entire grain kernel—bran (the fiber-rich outer layer), germ (the nutrient-dense core), and endosperm (the starchy middle). This complete package provides fiber, complex carbohydrates, protein, healthy fats, antioxidants, and numerous vitamins and minerals including B vitamins, iron, magnesium, and selenium.
- **Refined grains** have been processed to remove the bran and germ, leaving only the starchy endosperm. This processing strips away most of the fiber, protein, healthy fats, and micronutrients. White bread, white rice, and regular pasta are common examples.

"Whole wheat" versus "whole grain"—yes, there's a difference. "Whole wheat" refers to products made from the entire wheat kernel. "Whole grain" is the broader category that includes wheat and also oats, brown rice, quinoa, barley, and other grains in their complete form. Both are nutritionally superior to refined options, but whole grain gives you more variety and different nutrient profiles.

Why "Whole Wheat Pasta" Isn't the Same as "Whole Grains"

Here's where many people get confused: A product can be made from "whole wheat" and still be highly processed. Whole wheat pasta, for example, starts with the entire wheat kernel, but it's ground into flour, mixed with water, shaped, and dried. While it retains more nutrients than regular pasta, it's still a processed food that your body will digest more quickly than, say, intact wheat berries or steel-cut oats.

The closer a grain is to its natural, intact form, the better. Here's the hierarchy from least to most processed:

- **Intact whole grains:** Steel-cut oats, quinoa, brown rice, barley, farro, wheat berries
- **Minimally processed whole grains:** Rolled oats, bulgur wheat, whole grain breakfast cereals with few ingredients
- **More processed but still whole grain:** Whole wheat bread, whole wheat pasta, whole grain crackers
- **Refined grains:** White bread, white rice, regular pasta, most crackers and cereals

This doesn't mean that you should never eat whole wheat pasta; it's still a much better choice than regular pasta. But understand that even "healthy" processed foods don't provide the same steady energy and blood sugar control as intact whole grains do.

Understanding Carbohydrates: The Blood Sugar Story

David, a forty-eight-year-old accountant with type 2 diabetes, came to me frustrated by his poor blood sugar control. Despite following his endocrinologist's advice to limit his consumption of carbohydrates, his glucose readings remained erratic, with energy crashes and cravings that led to poor food choices. He was trying to avoid carbs completely but then would get so hungry that he'd end up eating whatever was easily available, usually something processed and high in sugar. His "low-carb" diet consisted of protein bars, processed low-carb products, and the occasional salad. The few carbohydrates he did consume came from highly refined sources that spiked his blood sugar level despite their limited quantity.

I explained that the issue wasn't carbohydrates themselves but the types of carbohydrates and how they're processed. Ultraprocessed foods, whether they're marketed as "low-carb" protein bars or regular cookies, disrupt blood sugar and hunger signals. Whole food carbohydrates, on the other hand, provide steady energy when eaten in appropriate portions.

We worked together to incorporate moderate portions of intact whole grains—quinoa, brown rice, and barley—into his meals, always paired with protein and healthy fat to further slow glucose absorption. I emphasized choosing the least processed versions: steel-cut oats instead of instant oatmeal, brown rice instead of white, and when he did have pasta, doing so as an occasional food rather than a daily staple.

David was skeptical but willing to try. Two weeks later, his glucose logs showed more stable readings throughout the day, fewer spikes, and importantly, fewer of the crashes that had previously triggered his poor food choices. His energy was steadier, and his cravings had diminished significantly. He'd never understood that there was such a difference between a serving of quinoa and a serving of white bread or that the degree of processing could matter as much as the type of grain.

Research consistently shows that whole grain consumption reduces the risk of developing heart disease, type 2 diabetes, and certain cancers. Most dietary guidelines recommend three to five servings daily, a target most Americans fall short of meeting. But here's what's important: These studies are comparing whole grains to refined grains and ultraprocessed foods, not to vegetable-based diets or other whole food patterns.

The takeaway *isn't* that you must eat grains to be healthy; it's that if you include grains in your diet, choosing whole, minimally processed ones provides significant health benefits over refined alternatives. For patients with celiac disease or nonceliac gluten sensitivity, numerous gluten-free whole grains exist, including rice, corn, quinoa, millet, buckwheat, and certified gluten-free oats. These provide the nutritional benefits of whole grains without triggering an immune response.

Practical Guidelines for Choosing and Using Whole Grains

Start with the least processed options when possible:

- Choose steel-cut oats over instant oatmeal.
- Choose brown rice, wild rice, or quinoa over white rice.
- Try intact grains such as farro, barley, or wheat berries in soups and salads.
- When choosing bread, look for those made with coarsely ground whole grains, visible seeds, and short ingredients lists.

When shopping, look beyond marketing claims such as "made with whole grains" and check ingredients lists carefully. Whole grains should appear first. The Whole Grain Stamp provides reliable identification, or look for specific language such as "100% whole grain" or "100% whole wheat." Remember that color alone isn't reliable; some brown bread contains caramel coloring rather than whole grains.

For more processed whole grain products, including whole wheat pasta or whole grain bread, treat them as transitional foods or occasional choices rather than daily staples. They're still better than refined versions, but they don't provide the same steady energy and blood sugar benefits as intact grains do. Portion awareness matters. Even whole grains are calorie dense. A serving is typically ½ cup cooked grains, one slice of bread, or ¼ cup dry cereal. Pair grains with vegetables, protein, and healthy fats to create balanced, satisfying meals.

I encourage my patients to experiment with various whole grains, preparation methods, and portion sizes while monitoring their energy levels, digestive comfort, and overall satisfaction. This personalized approach acknowledges that while some people thrive when including moderate amounts of intact whole grains in their diet, others feel better limiting them or avoiding them entirely. The key is to make informed choices based on your individual response and health goals, rather than following arbitrary rules about "good" and "bad" carbs.

Understanding these whole food principles becomes even more important when we consider the hazards of consumption in daily American life.

The Problem with Sugar and Processed Foods

The most common reason I see patients struggling with weight and blood sugar control is the modern American food landscape. It is full of highly processed foods—those with long ingredients lists containing items you can't easily pronounce—that disrupt our natural hunger and satiety cues. Food manufacturers employ teams of food scientists to create products with precisely calibrated combinations of sugar, salt, fat, and flavor enhancers that maximize consumers' cravings and consumption.

My patient Thomas was a classic victim of highly addictive foods. He came to see me for weight gain and concerning lab results showing prediabetes and elevated liver enzymes. When I asked about his eating habits, he described what seemed like a reasonable diet—morning coffee, a sandwich or salad for lunch, and a home-cooked dinner with his family. But as we explored further, a different picture emerged. His morning coffee was actually a venti caramel macchiato with extra syrup (over 40 grams of sugar). His typical sandwich came prepackaged from a deli. And while dinner was indeed home cooked, it was frequently preceded by tortilla chips and followed by dessert. Thomas was genuinely surprised when I calculated his sugar intake. Like many other patients, he didn't realize how much sugar was hidden in his daily choices. He also didn't understand how his brain was being hijacked by processed foods.

We worked together to gradually reshape his food choices. We began by finding less-processed alternatives to his sugar-laden coffee and identifying convenient but less-processed lunch options. We addressed the stress eating cycle with mindfulness practices and helped him recognize how certain foods triggered his overeating. Six months later, he had lost eighteen pounds without dieting. His liver enzymes had normalized and his blood sugar level had stabilized. Most important, he didn't feel deprived. He felt more in control of his hunger and satiety cues than he had in many years, which provided a renewed sense of calm.

Thomas's experience illustrates a fundamental truth: When you build your diet around whole foods—adequate protein for structure and satiety, fiber for digestive health and steady energy, healthy fats for brain and hormone function, and intact grains for sustained fuel—you naturally crowd out the processed foods that undermine your health. This isn't about perfection or restriction; it's about giving your body the tools it needs to regulate hunger, energy, and cravings naturally.

Rather than viewing foods as punishment or reward, I encourage my patients to think about their dietary choices on a spectrum, with whole, minimally processed foods forming the foundation. This isn't about moral virtue; it's about providing your body the tools it needs to function well. This doesn't mean never enjoying a cookie or a slice of pizza; it means building a nutritional foundation that will support your health while maintaining a flexible, compassionate relationship with food.

7

You Really Are What You Drink, Smoke, and Ingest

In the previous chapter, we explored how food is a foundational pillar of your health ecosystem. But your INPUTS extend far beyond what's on your plate. The substances we drink, inhale, and swallow all become part of your internal biochemistry. They influence your vital signs, lab test results, and how you feel. Your *relationship* with these inputs is informed by your biometric and biographic data.

Like food, these inputs can be nourishing to some and addictive to others. Also like food, certain substances carry social-emotional significance. Your coffee in the morning isn't just a jolt of caffeine; it might be the only ten minutes of solitude in your day. The drink after work isn't just ethanol entering your bloodstream; it's a ritual marking the transition from professional to personal time. The vape pen doesn't just carry nicotine that will bind to receptors; it might represent a momentary break from your noisy brain.

This complexity makes addressing problematic substance use particularly challenging. The typical medical approach often defaults to a binary view: Either you have a diagnosable addiction requiring abstinence, or you don't have a problem at all. But in my experience, the reality exists in the vast gray area between these extremes.

Understanding how your biographic data—your genetics, family history, mental health predispositions, and life circumstances—influences your relationship with various substances is crucial for making informed decisions. Some people can drink moderately without issue, while others have genetic variants that make alcohol addiction more likely. Some individuals metabolize caffeine quickly and can drink coffee late in the day, while others process it slowly and find that consuming caffeine in the afternoon disrupts their sleep. Your personal biology and life story matter enormously in determining what role, if any, different substances play in your health ecosystem.

The Biochemistry of Substance Use

To make informed decisions about what you put in your body, it helps to understand how a particular substance affects your biochemistry and how its effects show up in your medical data. While the full details would require a pharmacology textbook to explain, some basic principles can guide your thinking.

Most psychoactive substances—for example, alcohol, nicotine, caffeine, and cannabis—work by influencing neurotransmitter systems in your brain. They may increase the release of certain neurotransmitters, block their reuptake, mimic their effects, or interfere with their breakdown. These changes alter your mood, perception, energy levels, and cognitive function. The immediate effects may feel positive: relaxation from alcohol, alertness from caffeine, pain relief from opioids. But your body is constantly working toward homeostasis, or a balanced internal state. When repeatedly exposed to substances that alter this balance, your body makes compensatory adaptations.

These adaptations explain why the regular use of many substances leads to tolerance (needing to ingest more to achieve the same effect) and withdrawal symptoms when the substance is removed. They also explain why the apparent benefits of many substances diminish over time, while the negative effects accumulate—effects that often become visible in your lab work, blood pressure readings, sleep data, and other health metrics.

For example, alcohol initially increases GABA (Gamma-Aminobutyric Acid, the brain's primary calming neurotransmitter) activity in the brain, producing relaxation and reducing anxiety. But with regular use, your brain adapts by reducing its natural GABA receptors, leaving you more anxious when not drinking and requiring more alcohol to achieve the same relaxing effect. Meanwhile, its negative impacts on sleep quality, liver function, gut barrier integrity, and cancer risk continue to mount, showing up as elevated liver enzymes, disrupted sleep architecture on your fitness tracker, elevated blood pressure, and changes in inflammatory markers.

Similarly, while caffeine provides an energy boost by blocking adenosine receptors, regular use leads to the development of more adenosine receptors, resulting in increased fatigue when the caffeine wears off and the need for increasingly higher doses to achieve the same alertness effect. This shows up as disrupted sleep patterns, elevated resting heart rate, and sometimes increased anxiety scores on mental health assessments. This explains why taking a break from regularly used substances can provide valuable information about how they're affecting your health.

Alcohol: The Social Substance

Alcohol enjoys a privileged position in our society that few other substances share. It's legal, socially acceptable, and woven into American culture. Marketing firms have promoted concepts such as "wine moms," and retailers sell countless products bearing pithy sayings about alcohol. A glass of wine or beer is the go-to for many people to take the edge off after a hard day.

This normalization isn't accidental; it is cultivated by a multibillion-dollar industry and reinforced through social customs. The ubiquity of alcohol in our culture makes it easier to miss when consumption patterns become problematic. After all, if everyone around you drinks similarly, how can you know if your relationship with alcohol has crossed into unhealthy territory?

In the United States alone, approximately 14.5 percent of individuals aged twelve or older experienced a substance use disorder in the past year, with alcohol use disorder accounting for just over 5 percent. But genetic factors play a significant role in determining who develops a problematic relationship with alcohol. A family history of addiction, certain genetic variants affecting alcohol metabolism, and co-occurring mental health conditions all influence individual risk, making your biographic data crucial information for making decisions about your alcohol use.

My patient Nancy, a seventy-three-year-old retired office manager, exemplifies how alcohol problems can hide in plain sight. She had accumulated a long list of prescription medications from various specialists: Prilosec for heartburn from her gastroenterologist, Atenolol for high blood pressure from her cardiologist, and Prozac for depression from her psychiatrist. Despite those medications, she didn't feel well. Her lab work told a story her doctors hadn't connected: elevated liver enzymes, inflammatory markers, and disrupted sleep patterns. When I asked her about her alcohol use, she said that alcohol helped her relax at night. What had started as a glass of wine with dinner had escalated to a bottle most evenings, with earlier afternoon drinking on weekends.

Nancy didn't need a lecture from me about the harms of alcohol; she needed someone to help her see the connection between her evening ritual and her morning lab results. Over time, she was able to reduce her drinking; her reflux gradually went away, her blood pressure normalized, her mood improved, and her liver enzymes returned to normal ranges. We were able to taper down her prescription medications that previously had been treating the downstream effects of alcohol use.

When "Moderate" Drinking Isn't So Moderate

But what about people who consume alcohol who don't meet the criteria for problem drinking, alcohol dependence, or alcohol abuse? Just because you don't have a diagnosable alcohol problem doesn't mean that alcohol isn't affecting your health—and its effects are often clearly visible in your medical data.

Melissa, a forty-two-year-old marketing executive, came to me with complaints of poor sleep, constant fatigue, and increasing anxiety. On paper, her drinking habits wouldn't raise immediate alarm bells: a glass or two of wine most evenings, occasionally more on weekends with friends. She didn't meet the diagnostic criteria for alcohol use disorder. She never drank in the morning, never missed work due to drinking, and maintained successful relationships and a thriving career.

Yet her data told a different story. Her sleep tracker showed that even one glass of wine disrupted her sleep architecture, reducing her deep sleep by nearly 30 percent. Her anxiety spiked noticeably the morning after drinking two glasses of wine the night before, something we could track through her mood app and correlate with her heart rate variability data. And her digestive issues, which she had attributed to food sensitivities, followed a similar pattern in her symptom diary, worsening after alcohol consumption.

When I suggested a thirty-day break from alcohol to see how her body would respond, Melissa initially resisted. "It's just a glass of wine with dinner," she said. After reluctantly agreeing to a month without alcohol, she returned to my office with noticeable changes and notably improved biomarkers. Her sleep quality scores had improved dramatically, her morning anxiety had diminished (reflected in both her self-reports and her heart rate variability), and her digestive symptoms had dissipated. Her inflammatory markers had also decreased. "I didn't realize how much my evening wine was affecting me until I stopped," she admitted.

This illustrates a critical point: Substance use doesn't need to reach the threshold of clinical addiction to significantly impact your health. Melissa's moderate drinking, while socially acceptable and below medical diagnostic thresholds, was still a primary driver of her health complaints. Her body (and her data) was telling her something important.

Consider Michael, a fifty-two-year-old executive with recently diagnosed type 2 diabetes. When his hemoglobin A1C level was elevated at 8.2%, he was prescribed metformin; however, his blood sugar level remained poorly controlled. When I asked about his drinking habits, he admitted to having two beers most evenings, something he considered moderate consumption.

The connection between INPUTS and INFORMATICS was striking: His evening alcohol intake was spiking his blood sugar, interfering with his metformin, and disrupting his sleep, which further worsened his insulin resistance. His lab values weren't just about his diabetes; they reflected a complex interaction among his alcohol consumption, his medication, and his metabolic health. He cut back to one drink twice a week and moved it to earlier in the evening. Within two months, his A1C had dropped to 6.8% without changing his medication. "I had no idea my evening ritual was sabotaging my diabetes control," he told me. "I thought the problem was what I was eating, not what I was drinking."

This case illustrates how INPUTS directly affect INFORMATICS: Lab values such as A1C, liver enzymes, and lipid panels often reflect our consumption patterns as much as age and genetics can.

The True Cost of Alcohol

So how much alcohol is okay for you? Should you worry that your nightly glass of wine will cause cancer? Or that abstinence might somehow harm your health? The reality is more nuanced than headlines suggest. While some older studies suggested that there were cardiovascular benefits from moderate drinking, more recent research has called these findings into question, showing that even low levels of alcohol consumption increase the risk of developing certain cancers and other health problems.

The effects of alcohol extend far beyond the liver, showing up throughout your health ecosystem in ways that are often measurable before they're noticeable. Alcohol affects every organ in your body. From weight gain and insomnia to elevated blood pressure and increased cancer risk, its impacts accumulate over time. Even light drinking is associated with an increased risk of developing various cancers; this link is well established in the research. These risks may not be immediately apparent, but they show up in inflammatory markers, liver function tests, sleep quality metrics, and cardiovascular measurements.

Even though it may feel like a mood booster in the moment, with regular use, alcohol acts as a systemwide depressant. And by impairing judgment, it can lead to impulsivity regarding food, spending, relationships, and other behaviors. It can threaten jobs and family systems, often insidiously and gradually, without bringing about the dramatic "rock bottom" moments portrayed in movies. One of the most common patterns I see is the caffeine-to-wine "handoff": coffee in the morning, replaced by wine in the evening. This cycle creates a physiological pendulum swing between stimulation and sedation that disrupts natural energy patterns and can gradually erode health, showing up as disrupted cortisol rhythms, poor sleep architecture, and unstable mood patterns.

Why "How Much Do You Drink?" Is Often the Wrong Question

The traditional medical approach to alcohol focuses on the number of drinks people consume. This framing isn't just oversimplified; it can prevent people from honestly examining why they drink in the first place and how their individual biology responds to alcohol.

This is why I'm interested in my patients' *relationship* with alcohol as much as the quantity—and how their personal risk factors influence that relationship. This is what I explored with Nicole, a fifty-eight-year-old retired nurse who came to me with steadily rising cholesterol levels despite taking statins. Her LDL level was elevated at 160 mg/dL, her triglycerides well over 200 mg/dL.

What emerged was a story of complicated grief and genetic predisposition. Nicole's husband of thirty-two years had died suddenly from a heart attack eighteen months earlier. "Everyone keeps telling me I should be 'moving on' by now," she said during our second visit. "But I don't know how to be Nicole without being Tom's wife."

The grief had fundamentally altered her relationship with alcohol. During her marriage, she and Tom had shared a glass of wine with dinner once or twice a week. Now wine had become her primary companion in the evenings. It was the only thing that quieted the overwhelming silence of their empty house. "I know it's not healthy," she admitted, "but it's the only way I can fall asleep."

Nicole's drinking had escalated gradually and invisibly. What had started as a single glass to take the edge off had become a bottle most nights, consumed while looking through photo albums or watching their favorite TV shows. She wasn't drinking to celebrate or socialize; she was drinking to numb the profound ache of loss that haunted her.

Additionally, she had a family history of both addiction and cardiovascular disease—important biographical information that influenced both her response to alcohol and her cardiovascular risk. Her father had struggled with alcohol dependence, and both parents had died of heart disease.

The connections among Nicole's grief, alcohol use, genetic predisposition, and lab values were clear. Her case demonstrates how a biographical experience (sudden loss) had influenced her INPUTS (alcohol consumption as grief self-medication), which had then driven her INFORMATICS (cholesterol and triglyceride levels). Rather than turning to higher doses of statins, we addressed the root cause.

Working with Nicole required her to acknowledge that her grief wasn't a problem to be solved but a natural response to profound loss that had become complicated by isolation and guilt. We discussed grief counseling, and I connected her with a widow support group. Most important, we addressed her belief that missing Tom meant she was "stuck" or "doing grief wrong."

Within four months of beginning grief counseling, reducing her alcohol intake, and connecting with other widows who understood her experience, Nicole's lipid panel had improved significantly. More important, she began to understand that loving Tom and learning to live without him weren't mutually exclusive. "I'm not moving on from Tom," she told me. "I'm learning to carry him with me in a way that doesn't require wine to bear."

The question each of us should ask is about the impact of alcohol on our whole health ecosystem, including how our personal risk factors influence that impact. Specifically, how does alcohol affect your:

- Sleep, eating habits, and relationships? (behavioral health)
- Mood, anxiety, self-esteem, sense of self-regulation? (emotional health)
- Thoughts, judgment, impulsivity, memory? (cognitive health)
- Headaches, blood pressure, pulse rate, heart rhythm, blood sugar level, acid reflux, digestion, joint pains, neurological health? (physical health)
- Risk of developing dementia, diabetes, atrial fibrillation, sleep apnea, breast cancer, colon cancer, depression, substance use disorder? (medical risk—especially if you have a family history)
- Body weight, BMI, hemoglobin, hormone levels, liver function, glucose, hemoglobin A1C? (medical metrics)

Caffeine: Nature's Little Stimulant

America's most widely used psychoactive drug is part of the morning routine of most of us (including me). Caffeine has several well-documented health benefits supported by scientific research, but individual responses vary dramatically based on genetics and other factors.

By blocking adenosine receptors in the brain, caffeine reduces fatigue and improves alertness, concentration, and reaction time. Studies also show that it can enhance both short-term memory and sustained attention. It can improve endurance and reduce perceived exertion during exercise, particularly during aerobic activities. Regular caffeine consumption may boost your metabolic rate by 3 to 11 percent and increase your fat oxidation.

Large-scale studies have found associations between moderate caffeine intake and a reduced risk of developing several conditions such as type 2 diabetes, Parkinson's disease, Alzheimer's disease, and dementia. Contrary to earlier concerns, moderate caffeine intake (three to four cups of coffee daily) is associated with a reduced risk of developing heart disease and stroke in many studies, though individual responses vary significantly.

But here's where your biographic data matters enormously: Genetic variations in caffeine metabolism can make the difference between caffeine being helpful and being harmful for you. People with certain genetic variants metabolize caffeine slowly, meaning that even morning coffee can disrupt their sleep. Others process it quickly and can drink espresso after dinner without issue.

My patient Maggie, a seventy-five-year-old grandmother, discovered this the hard way when her Apple Watch alerted her to an elevated heart rate: 110 beats per minute. When I saw her in the office, her EKG revealed new atrial fibrillation, an irregular heart rhythm that increases the risk for stroke and congestive heart failure. When I asked her about her caffeine consumption, she admitted that she had been drinking three cups of coffee in the morning and iced tea in the afternoon to stay alert, following the advice that caffeine helped reduce dementia risk.

The problem was that she had both a family history of heart rhythm problems and likely slow caffeine metabolism; her biographic data thus made her particularly vulnerable to caffeine's cardiac effects. Her heart rate–monitoring data showed consistently elevated rates throughout the day, not just after coffee consumption, indicating that caffeine was staying in her system much longer than expected. We gradually reduced her caffeine intake to one morning cup, and within weeks, her heart rhythm returned to normal. Her sleep quality improved dramatically, which actually helped her alertness more than the extra caffeine had. For Maggie, less caffeine meant better overall function.

Similarly, my patient Sadie, a twenty-one-year-old college student, relied on Red Bull and energy drinks to stay alert in class. But her anxiety symptoms and insomnia were clearly linked to her caffeine intake in her symptom-tracking app. Her family history included anxiety disorders, making her more susceptible to caffeine's anxiogenic effects. When she switched to green tea and limited her intake to before 2:00 p.m., her anxiety scores decreased significantly and her sleep improved.

The key is understanding your individual response and moderating your caffeine intake accordingly. Most benefits are observed with the consumption of 200 to 400 milligrams (roughly two to four cups of coffee) daily, but your optimal dose may be much lower if you have slow metabolism, anxiety predisposition, or heart rhythm sensitivities. Pay attention to how caffeine affects your sleep data, heart rate, anxiety levels, and overall well-being rather than assuming that it's doing no harm.

Cannabis: A "Natural" High?

Perhaps nowhere is the relationship between biographic data and substance response more important than with cannabis. The rapid legalization of marijuana across the United States has been accompanied by wellness messaging that positions it as a natural solution for everything from anxiety and chronic pain to inflammation and insomnia. Cannabis dispensaries often resemble high-end wellness boutiques, creating a powerful impression of safety and wholesomeness.

What this messaging often overlooks is that cannabis has complex effects on the brain and body that vary dramatically among individuals. Your age, genetics, mental health history, and other medications all influence how you respond to cannabis. THC, the primary psychoactive component, affects cognitive function, motivation, memory, and coordination. Regular use can lead to tolerance, dependence, and in some vulnerable individuals—those with family histories of addiction or certain mental health conditions—addiction or psychosis.

Consider my patient Jae, a thirty-two-year-old software developer who came to me complaining of difficulty focusing at work. She had been a regular cannabis user since college, typically consuming a small amount each evening to relax after work. She didn't consider that problematic because she obtained it legally and never felt out of control while using it.

But her cognitive testing and sleep data revealed concerning patterns. Her cannabis use, while moderate by most standards, was affecting her sleep architecture and leaving her feeling foggy the next day. Her attention scores on cognitive assessments had gradually worsened over time, leading to problems with sustained focus at work. When her performance suffered, she sought help and was diagnosed with ADHD by a psychiatrist, who prescribed Adderall.

The stimulant medication initially improved her focus dramatically, but it also triggered anxiety and elevated her heart rate—effects clearly visible in her fitness tracker data. To manage those side effects, she had increased her cannabis use further, creating a cycle in which each substance was partially addressing problems caused by the other. Her family history included both ADHD and substance use disorders, making her particularly vulnerable to that pattern.

This isn't a story about cannabis inevitably being dangerous or Adderall being inappropriate; it's about how the "natural and safe" messaging around cannabis can lead people to discount its impact on their health—and how understanding your biographic helps predict your responses to it.

The same complexity emerged with Penny, a sixty-seven-year-old retired teacher whose chronic knee and back pain had worsened. When her massage therapist had warned her that prescription medications for arthritis were "unnatural" and would ruin her gut microbiome, Penny had switched to cannabis tinctures and edibles for pain relief instead.

Initially, her pain scores on her tracking app improved. But the temporary relief didn't stop her functional decline. She stopped gardening, abandoned her weekly walking group, and struggled to climb stairs. Her step count plummeted, her muscle mass decreased (visible in her body composition analysis), and her overall quality of life scores dropped significantly.

Six months later, she had found a more integrated approach: She used a low dose of Celebrex for inflammatory flares, continued her moderate cannabis use for sleep and breakthrough pain, and had completed a twelve-week physical therapy program that had improved her strength and function measurably. Her pain scores were better, but more important, her activity levels, muscle mass, and quality-of-life metrics had all improved.

Cannabis can be used responsibly and may provide benefits for many people. The problem is that it can also pose serious harm, particularly for those with certain biographic risk factors. Take my patient Robert, a fifty-seven-year-old architect who prided himself on his moderate use of marijuana. He told me that he consumed "just edibles" at night. At his annual physical, his liver enzymes were slightly elevated, and he mentioned occasional heartburn that woke him at night.

When I probed deeper, he admitted to using edibles specifically to avoid engaging with his son. It helped him disconnect emotionally, but it also led to late-night binge eating; the behavior he tracked in his food diary showed a clear correlation with his cannabis use. His liver ultrasound revealed fatty deposits, explaining his elevated enzymes, and his family history of diabetes put him at increased risk for metabolic complications.

Robert's nightly habit was causing measurable physical health problems and significant family conflict. After several conversations and a six-week break from cannabis coinciding with family therapy, his liver enzymes improved, his weight stabilized, and his relationship with his son strengthened. "I didn't realize how checked out I was in the evenings," he told me. His case demonstrates how even moderate substance use can become problematic when it serves as an emotional escape rather than a conscious choice—and how family history and other risk factors influence its effects.

Nicotine: The Addiction Amplifier

Of all the substances we've discussed so far, nicotine stands apart for its remarkable ability to create dependence. While caffeine, alcohol, and cannabis can all be habit forming, nicotine's addictive potential is in a different category entirely. Within seconds of inhalation, nicotine reaches the brain and triggers dopamine release in a way that can establish an addiction pattern after just a few exposures, especially in people with a genetic predisposition to it.

The health effects of smoking tobacco are unambiguous: It's the leading preventable cause of death globally, linked to cancer, heart disease, stroke, lung diseases, and diabetes. But the rise of vaping has created new complexities in how we think about nicotine use, harm reduction, and cessation approaches.

My patient Maya, a thirty-six-year-old graphic designer, exemplifies these complexities. She had smoked cigarettes since her teens and had tried quitting several times without success. Each failed attempt had reinforced her sense of shame and diminished her belief in her ability to change. Her morning cough was getting worse, her exercise capacity had declined, and her family history included her father's death from lung cancer at fifty-eight—important biographic information that made her continued smoking particularly concerning.

Rather than continuing the cycle of attempted total cessation followed by relapse, we discussed a harm reduction approach. She switched from cigarettes to a vaping device, eliminating the combustion products that cause much of smoking's health damage while still receiving nicotine. That wasn't an ideal end goal—vaping carries nonzero risks—but it was a significant harm reduction step that might eventually lead to further reduction or complete cessation.

The results were immediate and measurable. Her chronic cough disappeared within weeks, her exercise capacity improved (visible in her fitness tracker data), and her inflammatory markers decreased. Her lung function tests, while still below optimal, showed improvement for the first time in years. Most important for her long-term success, she regained a sense of agency over her health journey rather than feeling like a failure.

Maya's story illustrates several crucial points about nicotine and biographic data. Her father's lung cancer history meant that she had both a genetic susceptibility to nicotine addiction and an increased risk of developing smoking-related diseases. Her failed attempts to quit weren't personal failures; they reflected the neurobiological reality that nicotine addiction is among the most difficult to overcome, with relapse rates similar to those of heroin and cocaine.

The INFORMATICS in Maya's case were telling. Her initial lab work showed elevated inflammatory markers (C-reactive protein, white blood cell count) and evidence of oxidative stress. Her lung function tests revealed early COPD changes. Her fitness tracker data showed poor heart rate variability and reduced exercise tolerance. After she switched to vaping, these metrics gradually improved, though they remained worse than those of never smokers.

Six months later, Maya was ready for the next step: gradually reducing her nicotine concentration. We worked with her doctor to start nicotine replacement therapy, enabling her to further step down her dependence while maintaining the behavioral aspects of vaping that helped her manage stress and social situations.

This approach—meeting people where they are rather than demanding immediate perfection—often proves more successful than all-or-nothing cessation attempts. For people like Maya with a strong genetic predisposition to addiction, decades of established patterns, and high stress levels, gradual harm reduction may be more sustainable than abrupt cessation. However, it's crucial to understand that vaping isn't harmless. Emerging research suggests potential links to lung injury, cardiovascular effects, and unknown long-term consequences. For people who have never smoked, vaping represents pure risk with no benefit. But for established smokers, it can be a significant risk reduction strategy.

The key is understanding your individual risk profile. People with a family history of addiction, lung disease, or cardiovascular problems need to weigh the risks and benefits differently than those without these predispositions do. Your biographic data matters enormously when determining the safest approach to nicotine, whether aggressive cessation support, gradual reduction, harm reduction through vaping, or ongoing monitoring with minimal intervention.

The Integration of Inputs and Informatics

The delusion of harmless substance use isn't limited to cannabis. I've seen similar dynamics with:

- An executive whose infrequent evening vodka intake, combined with his genetic predisposition to atrial fibrillation, exacerbated his heart rhythm problems
- A college student whose Diet Coke consumption, given her family history of anxiety disorders, significantly worsened her panic attacks
- A retiree whose over-the-counter sleep aid use, combined with his age-related changes in medication metabolism, caused concerning memory problems
- A young professional whose vape use increased her baseline anxiety over time

In each case, the substance use itself might appear controlled and moderate, but it was functioning as a barrier to addressing underlying issues. True health requires an honest examination of not just what we use and how much but why we use what we use—and how our individual biology and life story influence our responses.

Your biographic data—family history, genetic predispositions, mental health patterns, age, medications, and life circumstances—provides crucial context for making decisions about substance use. They help predict who might benefit from moderate use as opposed to who needs complete abstinence. They explain why the same substance can affect people so differently. And they guide safer approaches when substances are used.

Your INFORMATICS—lab values, sleep data, heart rate patterns, mood tracking, cognitive assessments—provide objective feedback about how substances are actually affecting your health beyond how you feel subjectively. They can reveal problems before they become serious and confirm benefits when they're real.

The goal isn't perfect abstinence or perfectly optimized consumption. It's developing the capacity to make conscious, informed choices about what you put into your body based on understanding both your unique biology and the objective evidence about how these choices affect your health ecosystem.

This agency emerges from:

- **Self-awareness:** Understanding your unique patterns, triggers, and responses to different substances.
- **Knowledge:** Learning about how substances affect your body and mind specifically.
- **Honesty:** Being truthful with yourself about why you use what you use.
- **Data integration:** Using both subjective experience and objective health metrics to guide your decisions.
- **Flexibility:** Adjusting your approach based on changing circumstances and new information.
- **Support:** Seeking appropriate guidance when needed, whether from healthcare providers, peer support, or other resources.

For some people, this might mean moderate, occasional use of certain substances combined with abstinence from others. For others, complete abstinence from problematic substances while focusing on health-promoting inputs might be the right path. The key is that these decisions need to come from informed choice rather than unconscious patterns, cultural pressures, or misguided beliefs about what's "natural" or "safe."

By approaching substances with the same thoughtfulness you'd apply to any other aspect of your health and understanding how your personal biology influences your responses, you can reclaim power from both the substances themselves and the cultural narratives around them. You can reclaim agency over this crucial aspect of your health ecosystem, making decisions that reflect your unique health goals.

But these decisions don't happen in a vacuum. They're shaped by powerful cultural messages about what's "natural" versus "synthetic," what's "clean" versus "toxic," and what approaches are morally superior to others. These messages are often driven more by marketing than by science; they can also prevent you from making truly informed choices about all your inputs, from the supplements you take to the medications you need. In the next chapter, we'll explore how to navigate these false dichotomies and develop a more integrated approach to everything you put into your body.

8

Rethinking "Clean": Making Sense of Supplements and Diet Culture

The supplements aisle at your local pharmacy tells a story about how we think about health. Rows of brightly colored bottles promise everything from enhanced immunity to better sleep, from increased energy to weight loss, from sharper thinking to reduced stress. Their packaging often mimics that of prescription medications, lending them an air of scientific legitimacy. Meanwhile, behind the pharmacist's counter, actual prescription medications carry warning labels and require a doctor's supervision, despite often having more rigorous evidence behind them.

This physical separation reflects a deeper cultural divide: We've been taught to view "natural" substances as inherently safer and more virtuous than "synthetic" ones, "wellness" approaches as gentler than "medical" ones, and supplements as preferable to prescriptions. These beliefs shape not just what we buy but how we think about our bodies, our health choices, and even our moral worth.

But this divide is largely artificial and really more nuanced: Some natural substances are beneficial, others are harmful, and many are neutral. Some synthetic medications are lifesaving, others are overprescribed, and *most* require careful consideration of their benefits versus their risks. The source of a substance, whether from a laboratory or a plant, tells us little about its safety or effectiveness for your body and health goals.

What Is "Natural," and Why Do We Assume It's Better?

The appeal of "natural" products is deeply intuitive. We evolved in a natural world, so it makes sense that natural substances would be compatible with our bodies. This intuition is so strong that the word *natural* has become one of the most powerful marketing terms in health and wellness, triggering an automatic positive response in consumers.

But this intuition, while understandable, can lead us astray. The natural world is filled with toxins. Some of the most deadly substances known to humanity—from botulinum toxin to ricin to certain mushroom poisons—are entirely natural. Nature didn't evolve to keep us safe; it evolved through a competitive process in which many plants and animals developed toxins precisely to deter creatures like us from consuming them.

Consider my patient Elena, a forty-five-year-old teacher who came to me with laboratory evidence of liver damage. Her alanine aminotransferase (ALT) and aspartate aminotransferase (AST) blood levels were more than ten times the normal range. Initially, we suspected hepatitis or medication toxicity. But as we investigated, the culprit turned out to be a "natural" weight loss supplement containing green tea extract that she'd been taking for three months.

The supplement was marketed as "100% natural," "clinically proven," and "safe for daily use." What the marketing didn't mention was that concentrated green tea extract, particularly when taken on an empty stomach, can cause severe liver toxicity in susceptible individuals. Elena's genetic testing revealed that she had variants that made her particularly vulnerable to that reaction; her INFORMATICS made what was "natural" and harmless for others potentially life threatening for her.

There's no regulatory definition of "natural" on supplement labels. A product can contain highly processed ingredients and still claim to be natural if it originated from a plant or animal source, regardless of how many chemical processing steps it underwent. The kava supplement that causes liver damage is natural. The ephedra that can trigger heart attacks is natural. The aristolochic acid that causes kidney failure is natural.

Meanwhile, many lifesaving medications are derived from natural sources. Aspirin comes from willow bark. Many antibiotics originated from soil fungi. Digitalis, used for heart failure, comes from foxglove plants. The distinction isn't between natural and synthetic; it's between substances that have been rigorously tested for safety and efficacy and those that haven't.

The "Clean" Eating Mythology

Closely related to the nature fallacy is the concept of "clean" eating and living—the idea that our bodies are constantly under assault from mysterious poisons that can only be eliminated through special diets or detox programs. This messaging is particularly powerful because it taps into our legitimate concerns about environmental toxins and offers the illusion of control over them.

While it is true that ultra-processed foods are responsible in part for metabolic disease and liver dysfunction, the "clean" movement suggests that conventional agriculture, tap water, and modern life in general are poisoning us, and "cleansing" ourselves is necessary to restore purity to our bodies. But this framing fundamentally misrepresents human physiology.

If you have a functioning liver and two kidneys, you have a built-in, sophisticated detoxification system already! These organs have evolved over millions of years to handle environmental challenges. They don't need expensive supplements or elaborate cleanses to function; in fact, many detox products can actually interfere with these natural processes or stress the organs they claim to support.

My patient Derek, a thirty-eight-year-old marketing manager, spent nearly $400 monthly on various "detox" supplements after reading online that his chronic fatigue was due to "toxic overload." His regimen included milk thistle for liver support, activated charcoal for toxin binding, and a proprietary blend of herbs for "cellular cleansing."

When his fatigue persisted, we ran comprehensive tests that revealed the real culprits: severe vitamin D deficiency and sleep apnea. His expensive supplement regimen wasn't just ineffective; the activated charcoal was actually interfering with the absorption of other nutrients and potentially his medications. Within two months of treating his sleep apnea and correcting his vitamin D deficiency, Derek's energy levels normalized completely.

The toxins narrative is seductive because it offers a villain (mysterious poisonous substances) and a hero (clean products that can save you). But it also creates unnecessary anxiety and can prevent people from addressing real health issues. Instead of looking for new toxins to eliminate, I suggest focusing on supporting your body's *natural* detoxification systems through adequate sleep, regular movement, sufficient water intake, and nutrient-dense foods.

Wellness Culture: Inputs for *What*?

The wellness industry has lots of opinions about inputs. One month ashwagandha is being promoted as the solution to everything from stress to ADHD; the next it might be mushroom extracts, marine collagen, or rare Amazonian superfruits.

The result is a peculiar paradox: Many patients come to me more knowledgeable about obscure supplements than about the basic nutrition and lifestyle factors that have the most substantial evidence behind them. They can cite studies on rare adaptogenic herbs but haven't learned how to consume adequate protein throughout their day. They're taking expensive supplements to boost their energy but not addressing their chronic sleep deprivation or lack of physical activity.

My patient Jessica, a twenty-nine-year-old graphic designer, came to me feeling overwhelmed by conflicting health advice. She was taking twelve different supplements daily, following three Instagram wellness accounts with contradictory recommendations, and spending over $300 monthly on various products. Despite that investment, she felt constantly worried about whether she was doing enough for her health. "I see all these success stories," she told me, "and I feel like I'm failing."

Her comprehensive lab work was entirely normal. Her sleep tracker showed good-quality rest. Her diet, when we analyzed it, was actually quite balanced. The problem wasn't her health; it was her relationship with wellness culture. She was consuming content designed to make her feel inadequate so she would continue buying products and engaging with content.

We simplified her approach dramatically. She kept taking vitamin D (which her labs showed she needed) and a high-quality multivitamin, eliminated the other ten supplements, and unfollowed accounts that made her feel anxious about her health choices. Within a month, she reported feeling calmer, more confident about her health decisions, and significantly better about her bank account.

The Supplement Paradox: More Isn't Always More

The supplement industry operates in a regulatory gray zone that allows manufacturers to make sweeping claims with minimal supporting evidence. Unlike pharmaceuticals, which undergo rigorous testing for safety and efficacy before reaching the market, supplements fall under the Dietary Supplement Health and Education Act of 1994, which places the burden of proof on the FDA to show harm rather than requiring manufacturers to prove benefit.

This regulatory gap has real consequences. I regularly see patients experiencing side effects they don't connect to their supplements, delaying evidence-based treatments while pursuing supplement regimens, and incurring significant financial costs for products with minimal scientific support.

The wellness industry has masterfully positioned supplements as "natural" alternatives to "harsh" pharmaceuticals, ignoring both the potential risks of supplements and the natural origins of many medications. This false dichotomy prevents people from evaluating substances based on evidence rather than their origin story.

What makes this particularly concerning is how supplements can interact with prescription medications and other health conditions—interactions that often don't show up until problems occur. St. John's wort, commonly used for depression, can reduce the effectiveness of birth control pills, anticoagulants, and certain cancer drugs. Garlic supplements can increase bleeding risk when combined with blood thinners. High-dose calcium supplements have been linked to increased cardiovascular risks in some studies.

My patient Lee, a seventy-two-year-old retired engineer, came to me after a concerning episode in which his blood pressure had dropped dangerously low during a routine medical procedure. As we investigated, it turned out that he was taking a combination of prescription blood pressure medications and several "natural" supplements that also lower blood pressure, including aged garlic extract, hawthorn berry, and coenzyme Q10 (CoQ10). None of his specialists knew about his supplement regimen because he didn't consider supplements to be "real medicine."

The combination had created an additive effect that his doctors couldn't analyze because they didn't have complete information about his inputs. After we coordinated his care and adjusted both his prescriptions and his supplements with full knowledge of everything he was taking, his blood pressure stabilized at healthy levels without the dramatic swings.

A Framework for Making Decisions about Vitamins and Supplements

If you're considering taking supplements, here's an evidence-based approach.

1. **Identify the problem you're trying to address.** While targeted supplementation, such as iron for documented anemia or vitamin D for a deficiency of that vitamin, can be valuable, it's easier to take a pill than to address underlying issues. If you're low on energy, perhaps you need better sleep or more protein rather than B vitamins. If you're feeling stressed, maybe you need social connection or stress management techniques rather than adaptogenic herbs.
2. **Start with food.** Most nutrients are better absorbed from food sources, where they come packaged with fiber, phytonutrients, and cofactors that enhance their benefits. Before turning to supplements, consider whether dietary changes could address potential deficiencies.
3. **Use your INFORMATICS.** Get objective data through lab testing rather than guessing at deficiencies. Your genetics and medical history influence how you process supplements. What's safe for others may not be safe for you, and what helps others may not help you. Many people take supplements for problems they don't actually have while missing real deficiencies that could be easily identified and treated.
4. **Consider your biographic data.** The wellness marketing machine targets particular demographics by using algorithms on social media and making assumptions about your vulnerabilities and income based on what else you look at. Make sure you don't fall victim to one-size-fits-all marketing at the expense of your health.
5. **Cross-reference any supplements you take with all the prescription and non-prescription medications (such as antihistamines) that you are taking.** Many patients consider herbal remedies to be free of side effects because they're "natural," but plant-based products can interact dangerously with prescription medications. Always tell your healthcare providers about everything you're taking.
6. **Choose high-quality products from reputable manufacturers.** Look for supplements that have been tested by third-party organizations such as USP (US Pharmacopeia), NSF (National Science Foundation), or ConsumerLab. These certifications don't guarantee efficacy, but they do provide some assurance of quality and purity.

7. **Start with lower doses and monitor effects.** With supplements, more isn't necessarily better. Begin with the lowest effective dose and pay attention to how your body responds through both subjective experience and objective measures when possible.
8. **Periodically reassess your need to take a supplement.** Just because you started taking a supplement doesn't mean you need to continue it indefinitely. Regularly review your supplement regimen to ensure that it still matches your health needs and goals.

Remember that supplements are meant to supplement, not replace, a well-rounded diet. They're tools to be used thoughtfully when evidence supports their use in your specific situation.

Communication Advice: Talking with Your Doctor About Inputs

Whatever you take, please tell your doctor. When I see patients for the first time, I ask for a detailed list of all the substances they take—not just prescription medications but over-the-counter drugs, vitamins, herbal preparations, and other supplements. This comprehensive inventory is essential for several reasons.

First, some medications interact in ways that can cause harm or reduce their effectiveness. A patient taking a blood thinner such as warfarin, for example, needs to be careful about certain supplements such as fish oil and turmeric, which can increase bleeding risk. These interactions aren't theoretical; they can have serious clinical consequences.

Second, patients often overlook their use of nonprescription drugs, but they can be just as important. Frequent use of non-steroidal anti-inflammatory drugs (NSAIDs) such as ibuprofen can contribute to kidney disease or stomach ulcers. Regular use of antihistamines can impact cognition and cause drowsiness, especially in older adults. Decongestants such as pseudoephedrine raise blood pressure and can contribute to anxiety. Knowing what a patient takes regularly (even if they don't consider it to be a "real" medication) provides a more complete picture of their health.

Finally, this comprehensive inventory sometimes reveals patterns that wouldn't otherwise be apparent. I've had patients complain of persistent fatigue, only to discover that they were taking several supplements containing stimulants that were disrupting their sleep. Others experienced unexplained symptoms that resolved when we identified and discontinued supplements containing ingredients not disclosed on the label.

If your healthcare provider doesn't ask about your use of supplements, volunteer the information. It could be the missing piece of the puzzle in understanding your health concerns or preventing potential problems.

Common Interactions to Discuss

- Blood thinners + fish oil, turmeric, garlic supplements = increased bleeding risk
- Diabetes medications + cinnamon or chromium supplements = unpredictable blood sugar levels
- Blood pressure medications + licorice root or ephedra = dangerous BP changes
- Antidepressants + St. John's wort = reduced medication effectiveness
- Birth control + St. John's wort = reduced contraceptive effectiveness

Lab Values That May Reflect Hidden Inputs

- **Elevated liver enzymes:** Often due to NSAIDs or supplements such as green tea extract, kava, or multivitamins
- **Abnormal thyroid function:** Can be affected by biotin, kelp, or soy supplements
- **Unexpected electrolyte changes:** May be caused by sports drinks, protein powders, or "detox" supplements
- **Iron overload:** From taking iron supplements or multivitamins containing iron without known iron deficiency

- **Elevated blood pressure:** From consuming energy drinks, decongestants, or stimulant supplements

What to Bring to Appointments

- A complete list of supplements you are taking including dosages and frequency
- Bottles of the supplements or photos of the supplement labels
- A timeline of when symptoms started relative to the advent of taking new supplements
- Any changes in energy, sleep, or mood since starting new substances

The Prescription Medication Reality

Into this landscape of natural versus synthetic messaging comes perhaps the most moralized category of inputs: prescription medications. Despite being among the most rigorously tested substances we put into our bodies, prescription medications, particularly psychiatric medications, pain medications, and medications for chronic conditions, often carry a stigma that supplements don't. This stigma reflects our cultural narrative that needing to take medication represents personal failure, moral weakness, or a surrender of control to "Big Pharma." But this perspective ignores both the legitimate benefits of many medications and the complex factors that determine who needs pharmaceutical intervention.

Consider my patient Maria, a thirty-four-year-old accountant who had struggled with severe anxiety for years. She had tried meditation, therapy, dietary changes, exercise, and various supplements—all valuable approaches that helped to some degree but didn't fully address her symptoms. When her anxiety began interfering with her ability to work and maintain relationships, I suggested that we consider an antianxiety medication. "I don't want to be dependent on drugs," she told me. "I want to handle this naturally."

Maria's response reflects how deeply the natural/synthetic divide has penetrated our thinking about health. She was already "dependent" on her morning coffee, her evening wine, and several supplements, but she viewed those substances differently because of their origin stories rather than their effects on her brain chemistry. We spent time discussing how anxiety medications work and how they support the same neurotransmitter systems that meditation and therapy target, but more consistently and predictably for her particular brain chemistry. Maria's family history included several relatives with anxiety disorders, suggesting genetic factors that might make pharmaceutical support particularly beneficial for her.

After she started a low-dose SSRI alongside continuing her therapy and lifestyle approaches, her anxiety improved significantly. Her sleep quality increased, her work performance stabilized, and she was able to engage more fully in relationships. The medication didn't replace her other approaches; it supported them, creating the neurochemical stability that allowed her behavioral interventions to be more effective.

"I wish I hadn't waited so long," she told me six months later. She regretted having focused on doing things "naturally," as she had made herself suffer unnecessarily.

Prescription medications help control chronic conditions, relieve suffering, and extend both lifespan and quality of life. However, like all other powerful inputs, medications come with trade-offs. Side effects, drug interactions, and the risk of dependence or tolerance are real considerations that require honest discussions between patients and providers.

The key is to approach medications thoughtfully, understanding their proper role in your health ecosystem rather than either avoiding them when they're needed or relying on them exclusively when an integrated approach would serve you better. Sometimes the most "natural" thing you can do is support your body's chemistry with precisely targeted pharmaceutical intervention.

GLP-1 Drugs: A Case Study in How Society Moralizes Prescription Medications

Perhaps no recent medical development illustrates our conflicted relationship with pharmaceutical inputs better than GLP-1 agonist medications such as Ozempic, Wegovy, Mounjaro, and Zepbound. These drugs have sparked passionate debates and heightened ideological divides about how we treat obesity and overweight in this country.

Doctors, wellness influencers, and elected officials on both sides of the political spectrum seem to conceptualize obesity as *either* a problem of personal habits *or* a genetic problem whose victims have little control over their medical destiny. This framing pits willpower against drugs, nurture against nature, and is dangerously detached from reality.

This bias is evident in my own patients. They might praise someone who loses weight through strict dietary restriction for their discipline and commitment, whereas someone else who loses weight with the help of a GLP-1 medication is criticized for taking "the easy way out." Both approaches to weight loss affect brain chemistry, both require ongoing commitment, and both carry potential risks and benefits.

But what makes GLP-1 medications extraordinary isn't just the weight loss; they are sophisticated mind/body drugs that address physical and behavioral health in tandem. My patients on GLP-1s almost universally report changes in their habits involving food, not merely because they are less hungry but because these medications target the part of the brain where ruminations about food originate. The quieting of "food noise"—the constant mental calculations about eating that consume cognitive resources and emotional energy—can improve mental health in meaningful ways. I hear about it nearly every day.

Consider my patient Rachel, a forty-two-year-old attorney and mother of two who came to me having tried multiple approaches to weight management without success. She understood how to eat well and generally did—three meals a day, as discussed in chapter 6. But her inner dialogue about food and weight had become so overwhelming that she felt depressed and unsure of what to do next.

Rachel's struggle wasn't about willpower or lack of access to healthy foods; it was a neurobiological pattern that had become entrenched over decades. Her family history included multiple relatives with diabetes, addiction, and eating disorders. She also had an hour-long commute to and from work each day. Those biographic factors influenced her relationship with food, her ability to exercise, and her lack of success at losing weight through healthy eating alone.

After discussing all options, including continuing with behavioral approaches alone, we decided to try a GLP-1 medication. Her transformation went beyond weight loss. Within a few weeks, she reported a noticeable shift in her mental space. For the first time in her adult life, she wasn't constantly thinking about food. She ate when hungry, stopped when satisfied, and between meals, her brain was quiet.

The medication hadn't just affected her appetite; it had changed her relationship with food on a fundamental level. Her INFORMATICS reflected that change: improved insulin sensitivity, better lipid levels, reduced inflammatory markers, and stabilized mood scores. Her compulsive thoughts diminished, the constant calculations about what she "should" or "shouldn't" eat faded into the background, and food became fuel and occasional pleasure rather than an all-consuming obsession.

GLP-1 medications work through several mechanisms that make them unique among weight management approaches. They help regulate dopamine receptors in the brain, reducing compulsive thoughts about food and eating. They slow digestion, helping people experience genuine satiety, a sensation many people with disordered eating patterns have become detached from. They also improve insulin efficiency, helping the body process carbohydrates more effectively. For people with insulin resistance, this metabolic support isn't "cheating"; it's addressing an underlying biological dysfunction that makes weight management extremely difficult through behavioral approaches alone.

Of course, GLP-1 medications aren't appropriate for everyone and aren't without risks. They can cause significant gastrointestinal side effects, pose risks for people with certain medical conditions, and may contribute to muscle loss if not combined with adequate protein intake and resistance exercise. They're also expensive and require ongoing medical supervision.

Not everyone with weight problems needs a GLP-1 medication. Many of my patients need lunch—not Ozempic—to experience satiety. Some need a good therapist—not Ozempic—to work on body acceptance. Others need more time in their day—not Ozempic—to cook healthy meals to control their diabetes. Treating metabolic health is nuanced. The notion that any particular approach to health improvement is morally superior to others reflects our culture's deep-seated need to assign virtue and vice to medical treatments. This moralization doesn't just create unnecessary shame; it actively prevents people from accessing treatments that could significantly improve their health and quality of life.

Eating to Lose Weight: The Great Paradox

One of the most common barriers to sustainable weight loss is chronic daytime calorie restriction. Not eating during the day leads to overeating at night. Sarah, a thirty-eight-year-old marketing director, came to me concerned about weight gain and prediabetes. She wanted to try Ozempic. But when she described her eating habits, she explained that she was usually too busy to eat lunch. She told herself that she was being "good" by not eating during the day. Then, like clockwork, she would arrive home exhausted and ravenous around 7:00 p.m. She'd eat whatever was quick and convenient—often processed snacks while cooking—then have a large dinner followed by evening snacking while catching up on emails.

The pattern had started when she was in adolescence, when her mother had constantly been dieting and had made comments about her developing body. She had internalized the message that hunger should be ignored, lest she overeat and gain weight. As a result, she couldn't remember the last time she had felt hungry or full. Either she felt nothing until she was ravenous, or she ate until she was uncomfortably stuffed.

Sarah's body was doing exactly what our ancestors' bodies did during food scarcity: storing fat in preparation for the next famine. Her morning blood sugar level would spike as her body released stress hormones to compensate for missed meals. By evening, her insulin resistance had worsened, making her body more likely to store the calories consumed at night as fat. Her cholesterol numbers reflected that pattern of feast-and-famine eating.

Sarah's solution wasn't Ozempic or another strict diet; it was learning to recognize and respond to satiety cues throughout the day. We worked on her building regular eating habits: a protein-rich breakfast, a substantial lunch, and a moderate dinner. I encouraged her to tune in to her body's signals—what true hunger felt like, what comfortable fullness felt like—rather than adhering to the rigid rules etched into her subconscious. Within three months, her energy levels stabilized, her evening cravings diminished, and her lab numbers improved dramatically. Her cholesterol dropped 40 points simply by her redistributing her calories throughout the day. Sometimes the best prescription is self-compassion and permission to eat.

Beyond False Dichotomies: An Integrated Approach to Inputs

The most empowered approach to health inputs embraces both evidence-based medicine and personal preferences, finding the middle path between rigid orthodoxy and uncritical acceptance of marketing claims. This integration requires moving beyond the false dichotomies that dominate health discourse: natural versus synthetic, food versus medicine, wellness stamped versus doctor recommended. By moving beyond these artificial divisions, you can make informed decisions about what goes into your body. You can appreciate the legitimate benefits of both pharmaceutical innovations and traditional approaches while maintaining a healthy skepticism about exaggerated claims by any source.

The goal isn't to achieve perfect inputs; it's to develop consciousness about what you put into your body. It's understanding that everything you eat, drink, and ingest has consequences; that these consequences vary dramatically among individuals; and that the most effective approach often involves thoughtful integration of different strategies rather than rigid adherence to any single philosophy.

Some people will thrive with minimal pharmaceutical intervention, focusing on nutrition, movement, stress management, and targeted supplementation. Others will achieve their best health through combining these approaches with appropriate medications. Still others will find that their genetics, medical history, or life circumstances require more intensive pharmaceutical support to maintain their stability and well-being. None of these approaches is inherently superior to the others. What matters is finding the combination that supports your unique body, honors your values and preferences, and enables you to live with vitality and purpose.

This integrated approach recognizes that optimal health often requires various inputs working synergistically—that your morning medication might work better when combined with adequate sleep and stress management, that your supplement regimen might be more effective alongside proper nutrition, and that your dietary choices can influence how well your prescription medications work.

Most important, this approach can free you from the shame and anxiety that come with moralizing your health choices. Instead of judging yourself for needing medication, using supplements, or enjoying foods that aren't perfectly "clean," you can make conscious decisions based on evidence, personal experience, and your broader health goals.

Your body is neither a temple that must be kept pure nor a machine that can be optimized through the right combination of inputs; it's a complex, dynamic system that responds to various factors in ways that are partly predictable and partly individual. Treating it—and yourself—with both scientific rigor and compassionate flexibility is the path to sustainable health and genuine well-being.

KNOW YOURSELF, ADVOCATE FOR YOURSELF

Your INPUTS
Reflection and Action Guide

PART 1 Self-Reflection: Understanding Your INPUTS Landscape

Ready for more journaling? Let's go! Take some time to consider these questions about what goes into your body and how it affects your overall health.

INPUTS Inventory

- What foods, beverages, medications, supplements, and substances (legal or illicit) do you consume regularly?
- Which of these do you consider essential to your health and well-being? Why?
- How do various foods, beverages, or substances affect your energy, mood, sleep, or physical symptoms?

Your Relationship with Substances

For each input you listed, ask yourself:

- How often do I use it?
- What effects do I notice—both positive and negative?
- Why do I use it? (Be honest—is it habit, enjoyment, coping, social pressure, survival?)
- Have I tried going without it? If so, what happened?
- Does it align with my broader health goals?

Emotional and Cultural Context

- How do stress, emotions, or social situations influence what you consume?
- What rituals or habits have you developed around certain substances (morning coffee, evening wine, comfort foods)?
- How has your relationship with certain inputs changed throughout your life?
- Are you being honest with healthcare providers about your inputs and the purpose they serve?

Integration Across Quadrants

- How do your inputs affect your medical data and lab results (INFORMATICS quadrant)?
- How does your biometric data affect your inputs (e.g., high cholesterol and diet)? How does your biographic data affect your inputs (e.g., social isolation and alcohol use)?

Reclaiming Agency

- Where do you feel you have the most agency over your inputs? Where do you feel the least?
- What small, sustainable changes might better align your inputs with your overall health goals?
- Identify any substances you'd like to modify your relationship with—whether that means reduction, elimination, or simply more mindful use.

PART 2 Healthcare Conversations: Questions and Strategies for Medical Encounters

Questions to Ask Your Doctor

- "How might this [food/medication/supplement/substance] affect my lab data, symptoms, and risk for disease?"
- "Are there any evidence-based nutritional approaches that might improve my health condition?"
- "What do you suggest I eat in a day?"
- "Who in the public square can I trust when it comes to natural approaches to health?"
- "What supplements and vitamins do I absolutely need? Which ones might do harm?
- "Do you think I need to quit consuming X altogether, or is there a middle ground?"
- "Where could I get extra support for my [nutrition/supplement routine/behaviors around eating/substance use]?"

Communication Strategies

- Bring a complete list of everything you consume regularly (medications, supplements, alcohol, etc.).
- Discuss food patterns (e.g., "a day in the life" of your eating) rather than isolated examples.
- Ask about both benefits *and* risks of recommended treatments.
- Request specific guidance on timing of medications with meals and other medications.
- Ask for support structures and resources to make desired changes (e.g., apps, support groups, dietitians, therapists, health coaches).
- Be honest about your current relationship with food, alcohol, and everything you ingest, including any concerns or struggles.
- Request written care plans that include realistic, step-by-step approaches to dietary or substance changes.

Remember: The goal isn't judging yourself but achieving awareness. Whatever patterns you discover represent valuable information about your health ecosystem—data that can guide your next steps toward greater well-being and agency over what you put into your body.

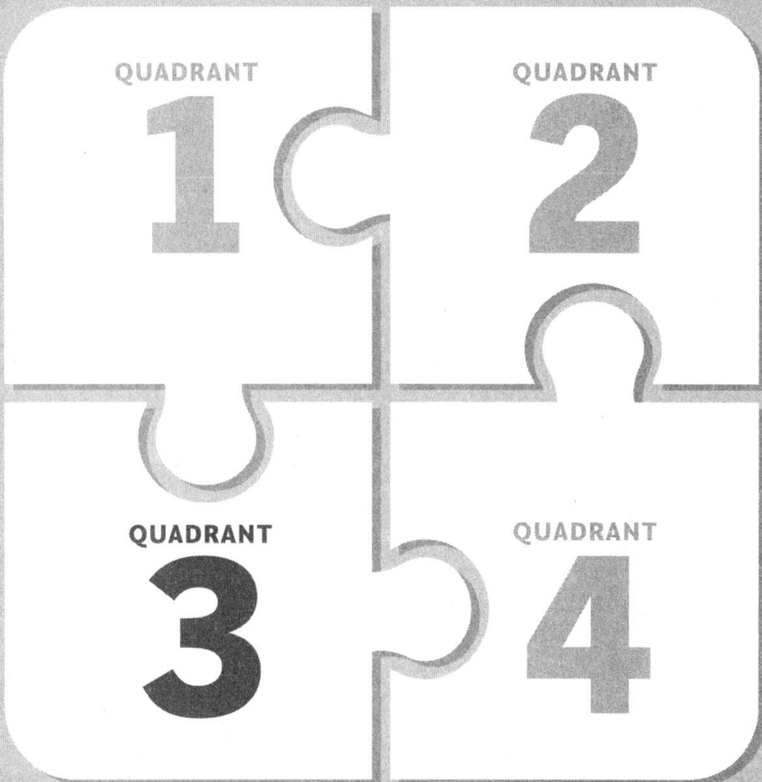

INFRASTRUCTURE

Your body is the vehicle that drives you through life. Unlike your car, you can't trade it in or upgrade to a newer model. The INFRASTRUCTURE quadrant encompasses your entire physical framework: your bones, muscles, tendons, fascia, and all the connective tissues that carry you through life.

This is where the rubber meets the road in your health ecosystem. Your infrastructure directly influences every lab value in your INFORMATICS quadrant: Regular movement can transform your cholesterol levels, blood sugar level, and blood pressure more dramatically than many medications can. It shapes your INPUTS, too: When you're in pain, you're more likely to reach for comfort food or skip meals entirely. When you feel strong and energetic, you make different choices about what you put into your body.

Yet most of us treat our cars better than we do our bodies. We change our car's oil regularly, rotate its tires, and respond immediately to unusual noises. But we ignore our body's maintenance signals until something breaks down catastrophically. We'll spend thousands of dollars on a gym membership we never use while neglecting the daily movement that keeps our joints healthy. We'll buy ergonomic chairs for work but spend hours hunched over our phone, ruining our posture.

Your physical infrastructure isn't just about preventing pain or staying mobile; it influences your energy levels, sleep quality, mood, and confidence. It determines whether you can play with your grandchildren, carry groceries without strain, or wake up feeling rested rather than stiff and achy. Ask anyone who's twisted an ankle, thrown out their back, or lives with a chronic disability how physical limitations affect every aspect of life.

In both conventional medicine and wellness culture, this quadrant is often oversimplified. Medicine tends to focus on fixing what's broken rather than maintaining what's working. Wellness culture promises quick transformations through extreme protocols that most people can't sustain. The reality is more complex: Your infrastructure needs consistent, intelligent attention throughout your lifetime, adapted to your changing circumstances, limitations, and goals.

Understanding your INFRASTRUCTURE means recognizing that movement is medicine, injury is information, and adaptation is strength. It means seeing your body not as a machine that should never break down but as a remarkable system that can heal itself, adapt, and even thrive within limitations when given proper care and attention.

By the end of this section, you'll understand how to be a good steward of your physical self—not through punishment or the pursuit of perfection but through sustainable practices that honor both your body's capabilities and its constraints.

Movement as Medicine

Regular physical activity may be the single most effective balm for every body system. Even modest amounts of movement can transform your laboratory values, vital signs, and overall health trajectory in ways that often outperform pharmaceutical interventions.

Consider my patient Richard, a sixty-two-year-old with high blood pressure, prediabetes, and elevated cholesterol. Like many patients, he arrived at his annual physical exam expecting to leave with prescriptions. While medication certainly has its place, I suggested that we first try a structured exercise program focused primarily on strength training with weights combined with brief cardiovascular intervals.

Richard was skeptical but willing to give it a shot. Three months later, his follow-up blood work told a remarkable story: His hemoglobin A1C had dropped from 6.4% to 5.7%, moving him out of the prediabetic range. His blood pressure had declined from 148/92 mmHg to 128/82 mmHg. His LDL ("bad" cholesterol) level had fallen by 15 points, while his HDL ("good" cholesterol) level had increased by 8 points. His triglyceride level had decreased by almost 40 percent. Those weren't just numbers on a page; they represented tangible improvements in Richard's health, achieved without a single prescription medication. The physiological magic of regular movement and weight-bearing workouts had transformed his metabolic profile and substantially reduced his risk of developing cardiovascular disease and diabetes.

Similarly, take Debra, a fifty-eight-year-old high school teacher whose blood pressure and hemoglobin A1C rose higher every time I saw her. She was taking the appropriate medications (Losartan for blood pressure, Metformin for type 2 diabetes), but she had repeatedly resisted exercising, admitting to me that she had always associated exercise with "punishment" for overeating. She admitted that not exercising felt strangely empowering, as if she were "giving the middle finger to my harsh inner critic." The problem was that her lack of movement only increased her cardiovascular risk factors.

So I helped her reframe exercise not as a weight loss tool (for most people, it isn't effective for weight loss) but as a way of honoring her body. She started slowly with a ballroom dance class once a week, reminding herself how much she loved moving to music. Over the course of a year, she hasn't lost any weight, but that wasn't the point. After she added thirty minutes of water aerobics three times per week, her blood pressure and diabetes tests normalized. She also felt more in control of her skeletal health (and inner critic) than ever before.

Both patients' stories illustrate how your INFRASTRUCTURE directly influences your INFORMATICS. This connection works both ways: Your medical data can guide your exercise decisions, while your physical activity reshapes your biomarkers in measurable ways.

Movement as Data: How Exercise Shows Up in Your INFORMATICS

Richard and Debra's cases aren't anomalies. If you need to be convinced of why regular exercise is not just good but transformative, consider this list of the systems that benefit from your moving your body.

- **Cardiovascular health:** Regular physical activity strengthens the heart muscle, improves circulation, reduces inflammation, and helps maintain healthy blood pressure. Even modest amounts of movement such as walking thirty minutes daily can reduce your cardiovascular disease risk by 30 to 40 percent.

- **Metabolic function:** Exercise improves metabolic efficiency. It enables your body to more effectively move sugar from your bloodstream to where it is needed most: your muscles and large organs. With exercise, your cells (and their mitochondria) do a better job of making energy and regulating your blood sugar level.
- **Immune system regulation:** Moderate exercise boosts immune function and reduces inflammation, helping the body resist infections and manage chronic inflammatory conditions. The anti-inflammatory effects of regular movement can be measured in reduced C-reactive protein and other inflammatory markers.
- **Brain health:** Physical activity increases blood flow to the brain, promotes the growth of new neurons and synapses, and enhances cognitive function. Regular exercisers demonstrate better memory, sharper thinking, and a reduced risk of developing dementia and other brain-based diseases compared with people who are sedentary.
- **Bone density:** Weight-bearing exercise stimulates bone formation, increasing bone mineral density and reducing fracture risk. This is especially crucial for women after menopause, when their declining estrogen levels accelerate bone loss.
- **Hormonal balance:** Exercise helps regulate cortisol, improves insulin function, optimizes thyroid hormones, and enhances testosterone and growth hormone production. These hormonal shifts benefit the entire body.
- **Mental health:** Some of the most compelling evidence for movement as medicine comes from studies on depression and anxiety— conditions that affect millions of Americans and that often exist beneath the surface of other health concerns.

The research supporting exercising to improve mental health is so robust that many psychiatrists now consider it a starting treatment for mild to moderate depression and anxiety. In some studies, regular physical activity has matched the effectiveness of antidepressant medications and does better at preventing a relapse in the long term.

My patient Ingrid had struggled with anxiety and mild depression for years, trying various medications with limited success. Her symptoms included persistent worry, sleep disturbances, low energy, and a general sense of heaviness that made everyday tasks feel overwhelming. When standard treatments provided only partial relief, we discussed adding regular exercise to her regimen.

Ingrid was initially resistant; the idea of exercise felt like another burden. "I can barely get through my day," she told me, unsure how she could find the energy for workouts. This is a common and entirely understandable reaction. Fatigue and low motivation are hallmarks of depression, creating a cruel cycle in which the very thing that might help feels impossible to initiate. We started with a gentle approach: five minutes of walking outdoors each day, with no pressure to go faster or farther. This minimal threshold eliminated the psychological barrier of "exercise" and allowed Ingrid to build a consistent habit. Gradually, as her body began to respond, she naturally extended her walks and eventually added brief strength training sessions using exercise bands. Within two months, she reported significant improvements in her mood, energy, and sleep quality.

Exercise works on several levels to create powerful mood-enhancing effects:

- **Neurotransmitter regulation:** Exercise stimulates the release of endorphins, serotonin, norepinephrine, and dopamine—the same brain chemicals targeted by many antidepressant medications. But unlike medications, exercise actually increases and improves the receptors of these important chemicals.
- **Stress hormone management:** Regular physical activity helps regulate the body's main hormone chain, the hypothalamic-pituitary-adrenal (HPA) axis, which governs stress hormone production. Over

time, this can reduce cortisol levels and improve the body's stress response.

- **Neurogenesis and brain plasticity:** Exercise promotes the growth of new neurons and connections, particularly in the hippocampus, an area that is often smaller in people with depression. It increases the production of brain-derived neurotrophic factor (BDNF), sometimes called "brain fertilizer," which supports the growth and resilience of brain neurons.
- **Inflammation reduction:** Physical activity has powerful anti-inflammatory effects, which may be particularly important given medicine's emerging understanding of depression as partly an inflammatory condition.
- **Improved sleep architecture:** Regular movement enhances sleep quality and duration, which further supports mood regulation and cognitive function.
- **Increased body awareness:** Movement reconnects people with their physical selves, counteracting the disembodiment that often accompanies depression and anxiety.

Exercise is not a blanket substitute for appropriate medication or therapy, when needed. But it does form an essential foundation for mental well-being, working synergistically with other treatments to optimize brain health.

Exercise as Personal Data: The Power of Tracking

One of the most compelling aspects of exercise as medicine is how quickly and measurably it transforms health metrics we can track on our own. Unlike many health interventions that require months to show effects—or that require medical encounters to see progress—regular movement shows up in our medical data within weeks and sometimes days. Wearable health trackers are popular for a reason: People like seeing the fruits of their labor. Of course, a health tracker can feel like an albatross to some, but tracking biometric data can provide powerful motivation and information about one's physiology.

Heart Rate Variability Improvements

Heart rate variability (HRV), the subtle variation in time between heartbeats, serves as a window into your autonomic nervous system's health. A higher HRV generally indicates better stress resilience and cardiovascular fitness. Regular exercise, particularly moderate aerobic activity, consistently improves HRV measurements within two to four weeks of starting a program.

My patient Callie, a forty-four-year-old accountant, began tracking her HRV using a wearable device when she started a walking program. Initially, her HRV averaged 28 milliseconds, which was in the lower range for her age group. After six weeks of thirty-minute daily walks, her average had increased to 35 milliseconds, indicating improved cardiovascular resilience and stress recovery. These changes occurred before she noticed significant improvements in her energy levels or sleep quality, demonstrating how the benefits of exercise can be measured before they're felt.

Sleep Quality Metrics

Modern sleep-tracking technology reveals how profoundly exercise affects sleep architecture. Regular exercisers typically show:

- 15 to 20 percent more deep sleep (the most restorative phase)
- Faster sleep onset (falling asleep more quickly)
- Fewer nighttime awakenings
- Better sleep efficiency (percentage of time spent in bed actually sleeping)

These improvements often appear within the first week of starting an exercise program and continue to enhance over time. The timing of exercise matters: Moderate activity earlier in the day promotes better sleep, while intense exercise close to bedtime can be disruptive.

Mood-Tracking Correlations

Perhaps nowhere is the exercise-data connection more immediate than with mood metrics. Apps that track mood, anxiety levels, and stress show consistent improvements in people who exercise regularly:

- Depression scores typically improve by 20 to 30 percent within four to six weeks.
- Anxiety levels decrease measurably after single exercise sessions.
- Stress resilience (the ability to bounce back from difficult days) improves progressively.
- Cognitive function tests show enhanced focus and memory.

My patient Malcolm discovered this connection accidentally when his fitness tracker began correlating his workout data with his mood surveys. He noticed that his anxiety scores were consistently lower on days when he exercised, even when his work stress remained high. That data helped him recognize exercise as an effective tool for managing his mental health, leading him to prioritize movement during particularly challenging periods.

The Power of Tracking

Understanding these data connections serves several purposes. First, it provides objective evidence of exercise benefits during periods when motivation wanes or progress feels slow. Second, it helps you optimize your program by showing you which types and timing of exercise produce the best biomarker improvements for your individual body. Third, it transforms exercise from a vague "should do" into a precise intervention with measurable health outcomes.

When patients can see their HRV improving and their sleep quality being enhanced, exercise becomes less about willpower and more about logical self-care. The data provides a bridge between the immediate effort of exercise and its long-term health benefits, making the investment feel more tangible and worthwhile.

This data-driven approach to exercise also helps healthcare providers and patients work together more effectively. Instead of generic recommendations to "exercise more," health-tracking devices can help develop specific programs targeted to improve particular biomarkers while tracking progress objectively. Your INFRASTRUCTURE directly informs your INFORMATICS, creating a powerful feedback loop that supports both motivation and optimization.

The Golden Triangle of Exercise: A Balanced Approach to Movement

The best kind of exercise is the exercise you will do. In an ideal world, my patients would get a combination of all three elements of what I call the "Golden Triangle": cardiovascular exercise, strength training, and flexibility work. Each component serves a unique function in maintaining your body's infrastructure, and together they create a synergy that exceeds what any single type of exercise can provide.

Doctors routinely recommend physical exercise to patients. But we often make several misguided assumptions: that patients want to exercise, know how to do it, and understand why it matters for their health. This is rarely the case. Many patients have been taught to view exercise as a nonspecific health obligation or a weight loss tool. They haven't been given the reasons why movement matters for their specific health needs, nor have they received a road map for developing a sustainable routine. The motivation to exercise often comes from a place of "shoulds" rather than genuine understanding or enjoyment.

Human physiology hasn't evolved much over the millennia. We are meant to roam the earth and move our bodies. The real question isn't whether you know that exercise is generally good for you; it is: How are you going to fit exercise into your actual life?

Cardiovascular Exercise: The Heart of the Matter

Cardiovascular exercise—anything that elevates your heart rate for a sustained period—delivers oxygen and nutrients throughout your body while strengthening your heart and lungs. Beyond the well-documented benefits for heart health and burning calories, regular cardio has profound effects on your brain chemistry, immune function, and metabolic health.

The beauty of cardiovascular exercise lies in its accessibility. While high-intensity interval training (HIIT) has gained popularity for its efficiency, don't underestimate the profound benefits of more moderate activities.

Walking deserves special recognition as perhaps the most underutilized yet powerful form of exercise available to most people. It enhances both brain and body function in ways we're only beginning to fully appreciate. Research has demonstrated that women who walked more than 4,400 steps daily (compared to sedentary women averaging about 2,700 steps) had a 41 percent lower mortality risk over a four-year study following 16,000 participants. Walking plays a vital role in managing weight, heart disease, high blood pressure, stress, anxiety, and depression.

Walking also boosts brain activity and creativity. It releases proteins beneficial to brain cells, and Stanford University researchers found that walking increases creative output by 60 percent as compared with sitting. It also aids recovery from injury and surgery, which is why hospitals now prioritize getting patients out of bed and moving as soon as possible. Most people can achieve these benefits by walking 6,000 to 8,000 steps daily.

How can you incorporate more walking into your day? Take the stairs rather than the elevator, park farther from your destination, conduct walking meetings, pace while on phone calls, listen to podcasts while walking, meet friends for walks instead of coffee, walk your children to school. The key is finding natural ways to get your feet moving throughout your day.

Other excellent cardiovascular options include:

- **Swimming:** Is gentle on joints while engaging the entire body
- **Cycling:** Is low impact with variable intensity options
- **Dancing:** Combines cardio with coordination and social benefits
- **Rowing:** Engages multiple muscle groups while being low impact
- **Elliptical training:** Provides foot-impact-free movement
- **Stair climbing:** Builds lower body strength while elevating heart rate
- **Tennis or pickleball:** Adds cognitive and social elements to physical activity

The best type of cardiovascular exercise for you is the one you will do consistently. I encourage patients to find activities they genuinely enjoy doing rather than forcing themselves into regimens they dread.

Strength Training: The Ticket to Healthy Aging

If cardiovascular exercise is about maintaining and improving our energy systems and circulation, strength training is about body structure and power. It's the architecture that supports everything else.

Despite persistent myths, strength training isn't just for bodybuilders or athletes. It's perhaps even more crucial for aging adults, sedentary individuals, and those managing chronic conditions. Resistance training—whether using body weight, bands, free weights, or machines—provides benefits that simply cannot be achieved through cardiovascular exercise alone.

If I could offer just one piece of advice to patients concerned about maintaining health and independence as they age, it would be this: Prioritize strength training. While cardiovascular exercise gets most of the attention in public health messaging, resistance training may be more crucial for healthy aging. Strength training preserves and builds muscle mass. After age thirty, we begin losing muscle at a rate of 3 to 5 percent per decade if we don't actively counteract this process. Consider my patient Margaret, who came to me at age seventy-two concerned about her increasing frailty. She had been diligent about her daily walks for decades but had never incorporated strength work into her exercise regimen. Despite her cardiovascular fitness, she was struggling with everyday tasks such as carrying groceries, getting up from low chairs, and climbing stairs.

For older adults, strength training makes the difference between maintaining independence and requiring assistance. Basic functional movements—rising from a chair, climbing stairs, carrying groceries—all depend on maintaining adequate muscle strength. Falls, a leading cause of injury and death among seniors, become less likely with regular strength training, which improves balance and reaction time.

Muscle mass loss can begin in our thirties, but it usually accelerates after we pass age sixty. There's even a name for loss of muscle as we age: sarcopenia. Age-related muscle loss increases our risk for type 2 diabetes, as well as high blood pressure and possibly heart disease and stroke. It can also contribute to obesity.

This pattern is extremely common. Many older adults do some form of aerobic activity but neglect resistance training, resulting in progressive muscle loss (sarcopenia) that dramatically impacts their quality of life and increases their fall risk. The consequences of this muscle loss extend far beyond functional limitations; sarcopenia is associated with insulin resistance, bone loss, increased inflammation, and even cognitive decline. For those of you who are not regular exercisers, the good news is that it is never too late to start. In fact, adding weightlifting or resistance training to your activities in your seventies and eighties can transform your skeletal health and your sense of agency over your body and mind. Caring for your physical container is caring for your overall health.

I suggested that Margaret start on a simple strength-training program focused on fundamental movement patterns: squatting, hinging, pushing, pulling, and carrying. Beginning with exercises using her own body weight and gradually adding resistance bands and light weights, she trained just twice weekly for thirty minutes per session. The changes over six months were remarkable. She regained the ability to rise easily from chairs, carry her shopping without assistance, and climb stairs without holding the railing. Her balance improved significantly, reducing her fall risk. Perhaps most unexpectedly, her chronic knee pain, which she had attributed to "old age," diminished substantially as her thigh muscles strengthened and supported her joints better.

Similarly, Mari, a fifty-one-year-old runner, came to me concerned about hip pain. She was in excellent cardiovascular shape, and her hip X-ray was completely normal. I moved her body around in my exam room. She had strong, developed quadriceps muscles, but when I tested the strength of her gluteal muscles (in lay terms, her butt muscles), she was weak. It turned out that her hip pain stemmed from inadequate firing of her left glute muscle, forcing the other stabilizing muscles around the hip to overcompensate, tighten, and cause pain. Her "back body" was essentially asleep as she powered through her runs using the brute force of her "front body." The solution wasn't more cardio; it was targeted physical therapy for her glutes, some careful stretching of her overworked quad muscles, and reassurance that her hip joints were just fine.

From a medical data perspective, strength training provides benefits that often surprise patients:

- **Metabolic enhancement:** Muscle tissue is metabolically active, burning calories even at rest. More muscle mass means better glucose regulation, improved insulin sensitivity, and a higher basal metabolic rate. For postmenopausal women in particular, strength training helps compensate for the metabolic slowdown that often accompanies hormonal changes. By strengthening muscles through resistance training, you're not just improving your appearance—you're building a metabolic engine that will continue to burn calories even at rest.
- **Hormonal optimization:** Resistance exercise stimulates the production of testosterone, growth hormone, and IGF-1, creating a more youthful hormonal profile that supports tissue repair, cognitive function, and overall vitality. These hormonal shifts help counteract the physical decline that typically occurs with aging.

- **Bone protection:** The mechanical forces created during strength training stimulate osteoblasts (bone-building cells) to lay down new bone tissue. This process provides the most effective defense against osteoporosis.
- **Inflammation reduction:** Regular resistance training reduces inflammatory markers such as C-reactive protein and interleukin-6, helping address the chronic low-grade inflammation that underlies many age-related diseases.
- **Improved body composition:** Strength training helps maintain or increase lean muscle tissue while reducing visceral fat (the dangerous fat around organs), even when total weight remains stable. This improved ratio of muscle to fat benefits several aspects of health.
- **Enhanced brain function:** Resistance exercise increases blood flow to the brain, promotes neurogenesis, and improves executive function. Recent research suggests that it may help protect areas of the brain that are vulnerable to age-related cognitive decline.

Other benefits of strength training include:

- **Improved joint stability:** Strengthening muscles around joints provides better support and reduces injury risk.
- **Reduced lower back pain:** Core strengthening often alleviates chronic back issues.
- **Improved balance and stability:** These lead to reduced fall risk, which is especially important as we age.
- **Enhanced functional capacity:** This makes everyday activities such as carrying groceries and climbing stairs easier.
- **Reduced arthritis symptoms:** Strengthening muscles around affected joints provides better support.
- **Enhanced mental health:** Resistance training correlates with reduced depression and anxiety symptoms.

What's remarkable about strength training is how little is required to see significant benefits. Two to three thirty-minute sessions per week, focusing on major muscle groups, can transform someone's functional capacity within months. I've seen patients in their eighties dramatically improve their quality of life by incorporating simple resistance exercises into their routines.

Effective strength training should include:

- Compound movements that work multiple muscle groups (squats, deadlifts, push-ups, rows)
- Progressive overload, gradually increasing resistance as strength improves
- Attention to form and technique to prevent injury
- Adequate recovery between sessions for the same muscle groups
- Exercises for all major muscle groups: legs, back, chest, shoulders, arms, and core

For beginners, I recommend starting with exercises that employ your own body weight to build strength, such as modified push-ups, squats, and lunges. As your strength improves, resistance bands provide an affordable, versatile next step. Whatever the modality, the key principle is to gradually increase resistance as the body adapts.

Flexibility and Mobility: The Often Neglected Element

The third side of our Golden Triangle is flexibility work with stretching, mobility exercises, and practices such as yoga or tai chi. This component is frequently overlooked, yet it connects and enhances the other two sides of the triangle.

Flexibility training maintains the range of motion in your joints and the elasticity of your muscles and connective tissues. Without adequate flexibility, you won't see the full benefits of your strength and endurance abilities. Lacking flexibility is like having a powerful engine in a car with wheels that can't turn properly.

It's not uncommon for me to see patients who have had X-rays and MRIs of their spine and who have even been offered spinal surgery, when the missing piece of the puzzle (and the key to improving their pain) is a basic stretching routine.

The benefits of flexibility training include:

- Reduced muscle tension and improved relaxation
- Decreased risk of muscle strains and joint injuries
- Improved posture and body alignment
- Enhanced coordination and balance
- Better blood circulation to muscles and joints
- Reduced postexercise soreness
- Improved range of motion in joints
- Decreased stiffness, particularly in aging individuals
- Reduced chronic pain due to conditions such as lower back problems
- Improved athletic performance across other activities

Flexibility work also serves as a powerful mind-body connection tool. Practices such as yoga combine stretching with breath awareness and mindfulness, creating a meditative quality that reduces stress hormones and promotes parasympathetic nervous system activation—the "rest and digest" state essential for recovery and healing.

For my patients with chronic pain, particularly back pain, a properly designed stretching regimen often provides more relief than medication does. The combination of improved tissue flexibility, enhanced body awareness, and reduced tension creates a virtuous cycle that interrupts pain patterns.

Effective flexibility training includes:

- **Dynamic stretching:** Moving through ranges of motion rather than holding static positions, ideal before other exercise

- **Static stretching:** Holding positions for thirty-plus seconds, best after exercise or as a stand-alone practice
- **PNF (proprioceptive neuromuscular facilitation):** An advanced technique alternating contraction and relaxation
- **Myofascial release:** The use of foam rollers or massage tools to release tissue restrictions
- **Mind-body practices such as yoga, Pilates, and tai chi:** Combine flexibility with other elements

Yoga, Pilates, and tai chi provide structured approaches to flexibility that incorporate elements of strength and balance as well. These mind-body practices create neurological patterns that improve coordination and proprioception—your awareness of your body in space—which becomes increasingly important for preventing falls as we age.

Bringing It All Together: A Balanced Approach

The Golden Triangle of exercise isn't about achieving perfection in any single area; it's about creating balance across all three. The synergy among cardiovascular conditioning, strength development, and flexibility enhancement creates a physical foundation that supports everything else in your health ecosystem.

For most people, I recommend something like this as a starting point:

- **Cardiovascular exercise:** Three to five sessions weekly, twenty to forty minutes each
- **Strength training:** Two to three sessions weekly, focusing on major muscle groups
- **Flexibility work:** Daily, even if just five to ten minutes

If time constraints make the above impossible, even small doses of each component will yield benefits. A ten-minute walk, a five-minute bodyweight circuit, and a few minutes of stretching are infinitely better than nothing.

Remember that exercise isn't just about medical metrics; it's about how it makes you feel. Pay attention to your mood, energy levels, and sleep quality as you incorporate more movement into your life. For many people, these immediate benefits provide more motivation than do long-term health outcomes.

Maintaining your physical health renders you more resilient in the face of illness and disease. From faster recovery times from the flu or COVID to better balance and coordination after suffering a stroke, keeping your physical container healthy is a smart investment.

When injuries, accidents, illnesses, or other events set back our physical health, it's also vital that we speak up about how those events are impacting our physical health. "No pain, no gain," "Suffer through it," "It's part of getting older," and many other mantras are outdated and untrue. Whether it is your knee, your back, or your pelvic floor, take the time to learn about how to integrate all your muscles and all your infrastructure into a more resilient physical body. Recovery following an event may look different; it also may be an opportunity to discover a better, more balanced you.

The Psychology of Exercise: Beyond Performance and Punishment

Many of my patients have described exercise as a chore, a punishment, or something they do even though they hate it. Others speak of past injuries from pushing too hard or trying to keep up with inappropriate programs. Still others confess that they avoid exercise entirely because they don't fit the athletic mold they believe is required. When framed this way, exercise easily becomes something to avoid rather than something that feels natural and nourishing. So for patients who are loath to get started, I suggest they begin slowly and with realistic, sustainable goals. The public health recommendation to get 150 minutes of moderate activity per week is aspirational; it doesn't have to be 150 minutes tomorrow. "Let's start with walking around the block," I often say, or "Try ten minutes a day or a yoga class once a week."

Exercise can also become psychologically addicting. My patient James exemplifies this struggle. A successful forty-eight-year-old executive, he approached fitness the way he approached his career: with intense drive and a focus on measurable achievement. His exercise consisted exclusively of high-intensity training sessions where he pushed himself to exhaustion, tracking every rep, set, and heart rate peak. He prided himself on taking "no days off."

But that approach had serious consequences. He suffered from frequent injuries, experienced persistent fatigue, and found himself dreading workouts. His cortisol levels were chronically elevated, disrupting his sleep and contributing to abdominal fat accumulation despite his intense training. Most tellingly, he admitted that he felt no joy in movement; it was a means to an end, a transaction.

We worked together to reframe his relationship with physical activity. Rather than viewing exercise as an arena for performance and achievement, we explored movement as a form of self-care and connection with his body. We incorporated more varied activities—hiking, recreational tennis, casual bike rides—into a more balanced strength program that emphasized quality over intensity.

The relationship with exercise can be complicated. So before you head out for your next walk, swim, or bike ride, take stock of how you think about movement and make sure that you're in charge of your routine—not the other way around.

Maintenance: How to Take Care of Your Skeleton as You Do Your Car

Most people would never consider driving their car for years without changing the oil, rotating the tires, or addressing unusual noises. Yet I have found that most people ignore their bodies' maintenance needs until something breaks down. Just like your Honda, your physical infrastructure requires regular care and attention to function optimally throughout your lifespan.

Preventive maintenance for your body involves several key practices:

- **Regular movement assessments:** Just as a mechanic might put your car onto a lift to check for problems beneath the surface, periodically assessing your fundamental movement patterns can reveal imbalances or restrictions before they cause pain or injury. Simple tests such as the ability to squat with your heels down, reach overhead without arching your back, or balance on one leg can provide valuable information about your movement health.

- **Addressing compensation patterns:** When one part of your body isn't working properly, other areas compensate, creating strain that eventually leads to breakdowns. These compensations rarely resolve on their own and typically require deliberate corrective strategies. Working with a knowledgeable professional such as a physical therapist, even when you're not in acute pain, can help identify and address these patterns before they cause problems.

- **Varied movement nutrition:** Just as your car needs different fluids and maintenance for different systems, your body needs varied movement "nutrition" to stay healthy. This includes strength work for muscles and bones, mobility practices for joints and connective tissue, cardiovascular activity for heart and circulatory health, balance and coordination challenges for neurological function, and restorative movements for recovery and stress management.

- **Respect for recovery:** Your body's adaptation to exercise occurs during rest, not during the activity itself. Adequate sleep, proper nutrition, stress management, and strategic recovery periods are essential components of structural health, not optional extras.

- **Environmental considerations:** The environments where you spend most of your time—your work setup, sleeping arrangements, frequently used furniture—profoundly impact your structural health. Optimizing these spaces to support good posture and movement patterns can prevent many common musculoskeletal problems.

Developing a maintenance mindset represents a fundamental shift in how many of us approach health. Rather than waiting for a breakdown and then seeking to repair your body, focus on creating resilient systems that can withstand the stresses of daily life while keeping your body in the best working order.

The care you provide your body now will determine the quality of your journey for decades to come. But even with the best maintenance, injuries and setbacks are inevitable. In the next chapter, we'll explore how to navigate these challenges while protecting the progress you've achieved.

When Injury Strikes

You're running to catch a bus when your foot catches on an uneven sidewalk. In an instant, your ankle rolls, pain flashes through your body, and you find yourself sitting on the concrete, stunned. Or perhaps it's more gradual: A persistent ache in your shoulder that you've ignored for months suddenly makes it impossible to reach for your coffee cup one morning.

When injury strikes, it rarely affects only the specific body part involved. As when we drop a stone in a pond, the ripples extend outward, influencing your entire health ecosystem in ways that might not be immediately obvious. You know the song "The hip bone is connected to the thigh bone . . ."? Well, it's true. When you injure your knee, your hip compensates. When your neck aches, your shoulder muscles adapt their position. These compensatory patterns can be protective; they can also create new problems if they persist long after the original injury has healed.

Skeletal problems can affect other aspects of your health as well. Your sleeping patterns change to accommodate the pain. Your food choices shift as cooking becomes more challenging. Your mood darkens as your favorite activities become temporarily impossible. Your relationships feel the strain as you require help with tasks you previously managed independently. In these moments, your body's infrastructure demands attention. The temporary breakdown of one component forces you to reckon with the interconnectedness of all aspects of your health. Everyone, regardless of age, needs to be concerned about their skeletal health. Injuries to our infrastructure can happen at any age, and responding to a serious injury is one of the most challenging undertakings for a patient.

While chapter 9 focused on exercise and maintenance, this chapter addresses what happens when things go wrong. We'll explore how to respond to injuries by understanding the connections between your infrastructure and the rest of your health ecosystem.

Muscles and Physical Functionality: When Imaging Data Doesn't Tell the Whole Story

A key part of understanding the musculoskeletal system is contained in the first part of the word, "musculo"—it is not simply about how our bones function but how our muscles, tendons, and ligaments interact and work to support and move our skeletons. Especially as we age, the medical focus is on joints and the need for surgical repairs. But sometimes it's the muscles and other soft tissues that need TLC.

Muscle Function Matters

When patients come to me with persistent pain, I've learned to look beyond their X-rays and MRIs to something that doesn't show up on imaging: how their muscles are functioning. Some of the most debilitating pain I see stems not from structural damage to bones or joints but from muscles that have essentially "forgotten" how to work properly.

Consider Samuel, a forty-two-year-old software developer who came to me with a decade-long history of debilitating back pain. His medical journey had begun in high school when he had injured his back during a wrestling match. At the time, his doctor had recommended what was then standard procedure: two weeks of bed rest. No rehabilitation, no strengthening exercises, no guidance on how to safely return to activity.

That approach had set Samuel up for years of chronic pain. As an adult, he had sought help from several orthopedic specialists when the pain had become unbearable. Each one had ordered X-rays, examined the images, and delivered the same verdict: "Your spine looks normal. There's nothing structurally wrong with your back."

Frustrated and desperate for relief, Samuel had turned to the wellness world. A chiropractor had diagnosed him with "chronic inflammation of the spine" and prescribed an extensive regimen of supplements: massive doses of turmeric extract, boswellia, systemic enzymes, high-dose vitamin D, a proprietary "bone-healing formula," kava for pain, and various "detoxifying" herbs that claimed to "pull inflammation from the spine."

By the time Samuel arrived at my office, he was taking fourteen different supplements daily. He looked exhausted, his pain was worse than ever, and his wallet was significantly lighter. More concerning were his lab results: His liver enzyme levels were three times the normal limit, his kidney function showed early signs of strain, his calcium level was dangerously high, and his vitamin D had reached a toxic level that put him at risk for cardiac arrhythmias. The very interventions that had been meant to heal him were creating new problems with his INFORMATICS.

What struck me most was that throughout the entire journey, no one had properly assessed Samuel's core strength or movement patterns. When I asked him to perform some simple functional movements, the real issue immediately became apparent: Years of compensatory movement had left his deep core muscles essentially "switched off." He had developed a pattern of relying entirely on his superficial back muscles for stability, creating constant strain and inflammation.

Samuel didn't need exotic supplements or spinal surgery; he needed help with his soft tissue INFRASTRUCTURE. This requires a functional assessment, not a photograph, to diagnose. Specifically, he needed to rebuild his foundation, especially the deep stabilizing muscles that should support his spine during movement. He didn't require a liver or kidney specialist to address his abnormal labs; he needed to stop the supplement regimen that was taxing those organs.

We developed a plan focusing on gradual core strengthening with a physical therapist specialized in spine rehabilitation. We discontinued all supplements except a basic multivitamin. Within two months, his lab values normalized. After six months of consistent work on his core stability, Samuel reported a 70 percent reduction in his pain levels. Most important, he restarted activities he'd long abandoned: hiking with his children, playing recreational basketball, even sleeping through the night.

In Samuel's case, the connections among his INFRASTRUCTURE (muscle-firing patterns), INFORMATICS (normal imaging results despite significant pain, abnormal lab tests), and INPUTS (harmful supplement regimen) highlight the importance of looking beyond standard medical tests to understand how these quadrants interact. His X-rays showed a structurally normal spine, yet he experienced debilitating pain. His labs revealed serious abnormalities due not to a disease process but to inappropriate interventions targeting a misunderstood problem.

Pain is only one piece of the puzzle, however. For certain medical conditions such as osteoporosis, addressing INFRASTRUCTURE problems can be superior to prescribing medications. Research clearly shows that bone density measurements (INFORMATICS) predict fracture risk, and these measurements can be improved by specific types of resistance training (INFRASTRUCTURE).

My patient Shelly's DEXA scan showed that she had osteoporosis. She was advised to take Fosamax, a prescription medication to help reduce fracture risk, but she had read bad reviews of it online. She and I discussed it in detail. We also discussed the fact that she hadn't engaged in regular exercise since she had been promoted at work ten years before. She noticed that her strength had decreased. Her weight had decreased due to low muscle mass. Her blood work showed that she was also low on vitamin D.

So we decided to push "pause" on the medication plan and instead focus on building back her muscle mass, tone, and strength—while optimizing her vitamin D level. I also noted that working on balance and coordination would help with her risk for falls, which would reduce the risk of fractures. Indeed, if she didn't fall, she was less likely to break something!

Many older women with osteoporosis dramatically improve their DEXA scan results through weight-bearing exercise rather than medication alone, showing how infrastructure interventions can directly affect medical data.

When Medicine Treats the MRI, Not the Patient

Modern imaging technology has revolutionized medical professionals' ability to peer inside the body without invasive procedures. MRIs, CT scans, X-rays, and ultrasounds provide invaluable information about structural issues that might otherwise remain hidden. Yet these technologies have also created a new problem: a tendency to treat the image rather than the patient.

Take Jane, a sixty-eight-year-old woman who had given up going to the pool to exercise because of debilitating hip pain. Her orthopedic doctor had stared at her hip MRI and told her she had osteoarthritis. He had instructed her to stop walking and start swimming instead; the pool would be a good low-impact alternative to her walking routine. But her hip pain only seemed to be worsening. She had been prescribed Meloxicam for pain but had stopped taking it when her cardiologist had scolded her for taking a medication that increased her blood pressure.

I asked her what else was going on. She laughed and reported, "Adding insult to injury, I've been having an increasing problem with bladder leakage and incontinence." As a clothing boutique owner, she had to interact closely with clients and even try on clothing, and she was worried about needing bulky bladder control pads. Her anxiety about incontinence had led her to stop attending the theater, as she was concerned that she would have to get up during the show or embarrass herself. She also reported having pain during sex, which was impacting her relationship with her husband. They had been going to couples counseling to try to deal with marital issues. All of that was making her feel old and hopeless.

It turned out that Jane's hip problem was a pelvic floor problem in disguise. The combination of age, three past pregnancies, and the lack of estrogen after menopause was causing weakness of the muscles that hold urine in, contract with sex, and support the pelvic organs. Her internal pelvic floor muscles were weak and misfiring. As a result, her hip joint was misaligned and inflamed. It wasn't the fault of the hip; it was the victim of her weak pelvic floor. The urogynecologist I referred Jane to figured out the problem "in ten minutes," Jane reported.

Jane's situation is a perfect example of how medicine's long-standing approach to women's health has frequently segmented issues. Internists and orthopedists aren't trained to ask women about pelvic floor muscles, yet they are crucial for hip and low back stability. Therapists don't usually ask about bladder issues. Gynecologists may not even ask about sex, not to mention connect it to nongynecological aspects of a woman's life.

The pelvic floor is made up of twenty-six separate muscles and is responsible for stabilizing not only the pelvic organs but also the bones of the pelvis and spine. The pelvic floor also assists with bowel and bladder control and is important for sexual function. Both men and women can have pelvic floor issues, but during pregnancy, hormonal changes and increased abdominal pressure stretch and weaken the pelvic floor muscles, reducing their ability to support the bladder, bowel, and uterus. A false assumption is that the only strategy that exists for dealing with pelvic floor issues is to do Kegel exercises. In fact, there are many types of therapies, and many people do not perform Kegels properly, so just doing the exercises by following a YouTube video, for example, does not necessarily yield results.

After evaluating Jane's symptoms, a physical therapist specializing in pelvic floor rehabilitation customized her program. In addition, I prescribed some vaginal estrogen to help her address pain and dryness during sex. The most important thing that I wanted her to know is that incontinence and pelvic floor issues are not a natural part of aging that must be quietly accepted. She had been right to speak up and seek treatment and not to dismiss her pelvic floor issues as something that could not be addressed. Our shared goal was to get her back into the pool and back to enjoying her life.

Jane's case illustrates a critical point: When structural issues arise, we must look beyond the obvious. An X-ray or MRI may show arthritis in the hip, but that doesn't mean the arthritis is the primary driver of symptoms. The human body is a complex system of interrelated parts, and dysfunction in one area can manifest itself as pain in another. This is particularly true of the intricate relationship between pelvic floor function and hip mechanics, especially in women who have been pregnant.

This holistic perspective becomes even more important when we consider how these physical issues ripple through the other health quadrants. Jane's hip pain and incontinence weren't just musculoskeletal problems; they affected her social connections, her intimate relationship with her husband, her mental health, and even her ability to maintain cardiovascular fitness through swimming. The solution wasn't just addressing the hip shown on the X-ray but understanding how her changing hormonal status (INFORMATICS quadrant) and pelvic floor function were contributing to her symptoms.

When Rehabilitation Beats Surgery

New hips, knees, and shoulders have been life changing for many of my patients. The ability to repair torn ACL ligaments and Achilles' tendons has kept people mobile and active, whereas in the past they might have been resigned to some level of disability. These surgeries have also helped with excruciating pain. But while a catastrophic injury or bone-on-bone arthritis can make surgery necessary, not every physical problem has a surgical fix. It's important to consider all the options when presented with physical pain, including that it's possible that you have not suffered a physical injury at all but instead that something else is going on.

Consider Ken, a former college athlete and current fitness "junkie" with lots of wear and tear on his skeleton who loves exercise for mental health reasons but who continuously gets hurt, then sees an orthopedist for every problem and gets scans and anti-inflammatory meds for short-term relief. He had been offered both a new hip and a new knee, but what he really needed wasn't a new joint; he needed a good physical therapist to understand the relationships among his hips, knees, and back and his old injuries.

When Ken first consulted me, he had spent over a year seeking treatment for various symptoms: hip pain that didn't resolve with minor cortisone shots, back pain that came and went, and knee pain that his orthopedist was convinced came from deterioration of his meniscus. Ken's X-rays and MRIs showed some arthritic changes in his hip and knee, which would have led many surgeons to conclude that his hip and knee joints were the cause of his pain. But when I observed him walking and had him perform various movements, I noticed something different: His pattern of movement suggested that his psoas muscle (a deep core muscle connecting the spine to the femur) was extremely tight on one side.

I referred him to a physical therapist who specialized in treating athletes, particularly those with complex, interrelated issues. After a thorough evaluation, the physical therapist confirmed my suspicion: Ken had significant imbalances in his core muscles. His psoas muscle was chronically contracted on one side, pulling his pelvis into an uneven position that placed stress on his hip, knee, and lower back. It wasn't a joint problem at all; it was a muscular issue creating joint symptoms.

With targeted physical therapy that addressed those muscle imbalances rather than just focusing on strengthening the affected joints, Ken's pain began to diminish. The therapist taught him exercises to release his tight muscle, strengthen his weakened core muscles, and improve his movement patterns. Within three months, he was hiking again without pain. His knee and hip joint replacement surgeries were canceled. What had been diagnosed as a structural problem requiring surgical intervention was actually a functional problem that responded to proper movement retraining.

Ken's situation highlights several common pitfalls in addressing musculoskeletal issues. First, the fragmentation of care—seeing specialists who focus on isolated body parts rather than the integrated system—can lead to missed connections. Second, the tendency to rely on imaging rather than functional assessment can result in treating the MRI instead of the person. Third, the preference for quick fixes (surgery, injections, medications) over comprehensive rehabilitation can address symptoms without resolving their underlying causes.

The modern healthcare system excels at acute interventions but often falls short with complex, chronic musculoskeletal issues that require nuanced understanding of movement patterns, compensation strategies, and the body's interconnected nature. This is why developing relationships with providers who take a whole person approach—and becoming an informed advocate for your own structural health—is so important. It's also why often a skilled physical therapist, not a surgeon, should provide a second opinion.

Ken's story illustrates how proper physical assessment can avoid unnecessary surgery. But it's equally important to recognize when surgery genuinely is the best option, rather than prolonging ineffective conservative treatment.

Is It Time for a New Joint? When Physical Therapy Isn't Enough

While many musculoskeletal problems can be resolved through conservative treatment, there are times when joint replacement surgery provides the best path forward. The key is to distinguish between cases in which surgery is offered prematurely and those in which delaying surgery causes more harm than benefit.

My patient Olivia exemplifies the latter situation. A sixty-seven-year-old retired librarian, she came to me with severe knee pain that had progressively worsened over five years. She could barely walk from her car to the grocery store entrance and had stopped attending her beloved book club because sitting for extended periods had become unbearable. Her sleep was disrupted by pain, and she'd become increasingly dependent on her adult daughter for basic errands.

"I don't trust orthopedic surgeons," she told me during our first appointment. "They just want to cut everyone open. There has to be another way."

I understood her skepticism. She'd heard the stories many patients share about people who had had surgery too quickly, who had experienced complications, or whose pain hadn't been fully resolved. Her distrust of the surgical approach had led her to pursue every conservative option available.

Over the previous three years, she had completed two courses of physical therapy with different therapists, tried acupuncture, received multiple corticosteroid injections, used prescribed anti-inflammatory medications (which she couldn't tolerate due to stomach irritation), explored various supplements, and even attempted several alternative therapies recommended by well-meaning friends. Each intervention had provided temporary relief at best, and some had provided no benefit at all.

When I examined Olivia's knee and reviewed her X-rays, the situation was clear: She had severe bone-on-bone arthritis in her right knee. The cartilage that should cushion the joint had essentially disappeared, leaving raw bone surfaces grinding against each other with every step. No amount of physical therapy, injections, or supplements could regenerate that missing cartilage.

I told her that I appreciated her preference for conservative treatment, but she'd reached the point where avoiding surgery was actually causing more harm than having it. Her quality of life had deteriorated significantly. The constant pain had led to depression and social isolation. More concerning, she was developing compensation patterns that were creating new problems. Her tendency to favor her painful right knee was causing her left knee to ache from overuse, and her altered gait was contributing to lower back pain. The longer she delayed surgery, the more challenging her recovery would become.

After extensive discussion and consultation with an orthopedic surgeon I trust, Olivia reluctantly agreed to proceed with total knee replacement surgery. Three months later, she was walking distances she hadn't managed in years. Six months postsurgery, she had returned to her book club and was taking daily walks around her neighborhood. A year later, she told me that it was one of the best decisions she'd ever made. "I wish I hadn't waited so long," she admitted. "I was so focused on avoiding surgery that I forgot I was avoiding life."

Olivia's case illustrates an important principle: While conservative treatment should generally be attempted first, there's a point where continuing to delay appropriate surgery becomes counterproductive. The goal isn't to avoid surgery at all costs; it's to ensure that it is truly necessary and that the timing will optimize the outcome.

Are You Ready for a New Joint?

There's rarely a "perfect" time for joint replacement surgery, but in my experience, people often wait too long rather than moving too quickly. Here are some signs that it may be time to seriously consider surgery.

Functional Limitations

- Your pain significantly limits your daily activities (walking, taking stairs, sleeping).
- You've stopped doing activities you enjoy because of joint pain.
- You need assistance with basic tasks due to joint limitations.
- Pain medications are required for basic function but cause unacceptable side effects.

Conservative Treatment Failure

- Multiple courses of appropriate physical therapy haven't provided lasting relief.
- Injections provide only temporary benefit (less than three to four months).

- Anti-inflammatory medications are ineffective or can't be tolerated.
- Your pain continues to worsen despite optimal conservative care.

Quality-of-Life Impact

- Joint pain is affecting your mood, sleep, or relationships.
- You're avoiding social activities due to pain or mobility concerns.
- Fear of pain is making you increasingly sedentary.
- Your dependence on others is increasing due to joint limitations.

Optimal Timing Considerations

- You're healthy enough to tolerate surgery and anesthesia.
- You have adequate support for a recovery period.
- You're motivated to participate in postsurgical rehabilitation.
- Any other health conditions you may have are well managed.

Signs That You May Be Waiting Too Long

- You're developing compensation patterns that create new problems.
- Your overall fitness is declining due to inactivity.
- You are suffering from depression or anxiety related to your pain and limitations.
- Your family relationships are being strained by your increasing dependence.

I often tell patients that getting a new joint is like renovating your kitchen: You don't want to do it, the process is disruptive, but you're almost always happy afterward. The key is to time the surgery when you're healthy enough to have a good outcome and before the joint problem creates additional complications.

Remember: Joint replacement isn't about returning to your twenty-year-old self; it's about reclaiming function and reducing pain so you can engage in the activities that matter most to you.

Injury as Proof of the Inseparability of Physical and Emotional Health

Physical injury doesn't just impact your body; it profoundly affects your psychological state as well. The bidirectional relationship between physical pain and mental health creates feedback loops that can either accelerate healing or trap you in cycles of suffering.

Take my patient Cathy, who underwent knee replacement surgery after years of progressive osteoarthritis. The surgery itself went well, but during her recovery, Cathy reported low moods, a diminished interest in previously enjoyable activities, difficulty concentrating, and fatigue—all classic symptoms of a depressive episode. Her original primary care doctor prescribed an antidepressant, assuming that her symptoms reflected a psychological reaction to her temporary disability.

When Cathy came to see me for a second opinion, I asked her about her post-operative recovery process. What emerged was a gap in her care. She had been discharged from physical therapy once she had achieved basic functional goals. No one had guided her through the transition from rehabilitation exercises to normal physical activity. Without guidance on how to safely return to modified versions of her favorite activities, she had defaulted to a sedentary lifestyle that had fed her sense of loss and disconnection.

I connected her with a physical therapist specializing in return-to-activity programs and a recreational therapist who could help her adapt her favorite hobbies, such as exploring local nature trails, to accommodate her new knee. We also addressed her fear of reinjury through gradual exposure to short hikes and education about her new joint's capabilities and limitations. Within two months, she had resumed modified versions of her favorite activities and her mood improved dramatically.

Similarly, physical pain and serious skeletal limitations often reflect psychological states; a person with chronic neck and shoulder tension may be literally "carrying the weight of the world" on their shoulders. Muscles can become so tight that they cause serious disability. Conversely, posture and movement directly influence emotional state and cognitive function, a phenomenon clearly demonstrated in research on "embodied cognition."

My patient Sophia experienced this connection firsthand when addressing her anxiety. Traditional therapy had helped her recognize negative thought patterns such as catastrophizing and obsessing over conversations with colleagues at work, but she continued to experience physical manifestations of anxiety: radiating pain and tingling from her neck to her right hand and fingers. Fear that she might have a serious nerve problem made her even more anxious. When I examined her neurologically, it was clear that she had a pinched nerve in her neck and that she wasn't going to get better with therapy and pain medications alone. When we added specific movement practices focused on diaphragmatic breathing and releasing chronically contracted muscles, her anxiety symptoms decreased, and her hand stopped tingling. That physical intervention helped interrupt the cycles of anxiety. With less anxiety, her muscles finally began to unlock.

These examples highlight a crucial principle: When injury strikes, treating only the physical structure or only the psychological response is insufficient. We must address both simultaneously, recognizing their profound interconnection. Pain affects mood, sleep, and cognitive function; psychological state influences pain perception, movement patterns, and healing capacity. Neither exists in isolation.

Building Resilience Through Recovery

Injury can be profoundly disruptive, but it also presents an opportunity to rebuild your relationship with your body in ways that create greater resilience and awareness. Many of my patients report that recovering from injury, while challenging, taught them valuable lessons about their bodies and health that they wouldn't have learned otherwise.

The recovery process often requires relearning movement patterns that were previously automatic, bringing conscious attention to habitual behaviors that may have contributed to the original injury. This heightened awareness can extend beyond the injured area, improving overall body mechanics, posture, and movement quality. Patients who embrace this process often emerge with a more integrated understanding of their physical capabilities and limitations.

Recovery also provides an opportunity to reassess priorities and practices across all health quadrants. When injury forces you to temporarily abandon certain activities, it creates space to explore new inputs, movement patterns, and self-care practices. The martial artist who can't train due to a shoulder injury might discover meditative practices that enhance their mental game. The runner sidelined by plantar fasciitis might explore swimming or cycling, developing new skills and cross-training benefits that will serve them even after they return to running.

Most important, successfully navigating injury recovery builds confidence in your body's capacity to heal and adapt. This resilience, the knowledge that you can overcome physical challenges, becomes a resource you carry forward, reducing your fear when future setbacks occur.

How Inputs Affect Recovery and Repair

Specific nutrients play critical roles in tissue repair. Protein provides the building blocks for rebuilding damaged tissues. Vitamin C is essential for collagen synthesis. Zinc supports immune function and wound healing. Vitamin D and calcium are critical for bone health. Omega-3 fatty acids help modulate inflammation. Recovery from injury may require temporary adjustments to nutritional intake to support healing processes.

Hydration status directly affects tissue health and healing capacity. Dehydrated tissues have reduced elasticity and are more prone to further injury. Fascia, the connective tissue that surrounds and connects muscles, organs, and other structures, is particularly sensitive to hydration status. Well-hydrated fascia moves smoothly; dehydrated fascia becomes sticky and restricted, potentially creating or exacerbating pain.

Cigarette smoking is known to interfere with wound healing. The excessive use of alcohol can weaken muscles and hamper recovery from skeletal injuries. Caffeine, when used in high quantifies, can increase muscle tension, trigger a spike in stress hormones, and disrupt sleep—all of which can prevent healing.

My patient Bernie, a thirty-four-year-old construction worker, learned that lesson the hard way after suffering a severe ankle fracture that required surgical repair. His initial recovery was progressing normally until week four, when his healing seemed to stall. His incision wasn't healing properly, he was experiencing more pain than expected, and his energy level was extremely low.

When I reviewed Bernie's typical day, a concerning pattern emerged. He was surviving primarily on energy drinks, fast food, and whatever his girlfriend could bring him during her lunch break. His protein intake was minimal at a mere 30 grams per day when he needed closer to 100 grams for optimal tissue repair. He was drinking little water but consuming multiple energy drinks daily, creating a cycle of dehydration and caffeine crashes that disrupted his sleep.

Most problematically, he was using his prescribed pain medication inconsistently, then compensating with alcohol in the evenings to "take the edge off." That combination was interfering with both his sleep quality and his body's natural healing processes. We made targeted changes to support his recovery: increasing his protein intake to 25 to 30 grams per meal through simple options such as Greek yogurt, protein shakes, and precooked chicken strips; replacing energy drinks with water and limiting caffeine to morning hours only; eliminating alcohol completely during his recovery period; and adding a vitamin C supplement and zinc to support collagen synthesis and wound healing.

Within two weeks of his adjusting his inputs, Bernie's incision finally began healing properly, his energy improved significantly, and his pain level decreased to the point where he could reduce his pain medication. His orthopedic surgeon was impressed with how quickly his bone healing progressed once his nutrition was optimized.

"I had no idea that what I was eating could affect whether my bone would heal," Bernie told me at his follow-up visit. Hiss experience illustrates how dramatically inputs can influence recovery outcomes. His body was trying to rebuild damaged tissue while being starved of the raw materials it needed for repair. No amount of rest or medical intervention could compensate for inadequate protein intake, chronic dehydration, and substances that interfered with the healing process.

Your physical infrastructure, your medical data, and what you consume continuously inform one another, creating feedback loops that can either support or undermine your health. Understanding these connections can make you a better consumer of healthcare and a smarter advocate for your health.

The Path Forward: Becoming Your Own Structural Detective

When injury strikes, becoming an informed advocate for your structural health is essential. Here are some strategies to navigate the recovery process effectively.

- **Seek root causes, not just symptom relief.** Pain is a signal, not the problem itself. Work with healthcare providers who will investigate why pain is occurring, not just how to mask it. This might mean looking beyond the pain site to movement patterns, postural habits, prior injuries, or even seemingly unrelated issues in other body systems.
- **Question single-factor explanations.** Be skeptical of providers who attribute complex pain patterns solely to age, weight, genetics, or structural findings on imaging. While these factors may contribute, they rarely tell the complete story.

- **Find providers who treat people, not scans.** Imaging findings often correlate poorly with symptoms. Many people with severe arthritis on X-rays have no pain, while others with minimal imaging abnormalities experience significant discomfort. Look for providers who base treatment decisions on your functional limitations and goals, not just what appears on scans.
- **Prioritize functional assessment over diagnostic labels.** Understanding how your body moves and where restrictions occur provides more actionable information than a diagnostic label alone. Work with practitioners who are skilled in movement assessment, not just tissue evaluation.
- **Explore regional interdependence.** The body works as an integrated system. Issues in one area often affect seemingly unrelated regions through kinetic chains and fascial connections. Addressing your knee pain might require attention to hip or ankle function; shoulder problems might connect to neck or thoracic spine mobility.
- **Build a collaborative team.** Different providers bring different expertise. Physical therapists understand movement patterns and exercise progression. Physicians can address underlying medical conditions and medication management. Massage therapists can address fascial restrictions. Mental health professionals can help with the psychological aspects of pain and recovery. Creating a team approach, with you as the CEO, often yields better results than relying on a single provider.
- **Track function, not just pain.** Focus your recovery goals on what you want to do, not just symptom reduction. Whether it's returning to a specific sport, playing with your grandchildren, or maintaining your independence in daily activities, function-focused goals provide more meaningful markers of progress than pain scales alone.
- **Respect healing timelines.** Different tissues heal at different rates. A muscle strain may resolve in weeks, while a tendon injury often takes months to heal. Bone healing follows predictable stages that

can't be rushed. Understanding tissue-specific recovery timelines helps set realistic expectations and prevents the frustration of perceived "slow" progress.

- **Address the whole health ecosystem.** Optimize your sleep, nutrition, stress management, and social support alongside physical rehabilitation. These factors significantly influence recovery timelines and outcomes.
- **Cultivate body awareness.** Develop the ability to distinguish between productive discomfort (the temporary strain of appropriate rehabilitation exercises) and warning pain (signals of potential reinjury or excessive loading). This discernment is essential for navigating the recovery process safely.

By approaching injury recovery with this comprehensive, detective-like mindset, you can transform a potentially frustrating experience into an opportunity for greater body understanding and long-term resilience. Remember, the goal isn't just to return to your previous function but to rebuild in ways that will reduce future injury risk and enhance your overall structural health.

In the next chapter, we'll explore how these principles extend into situations of more permanent disability, examining how to maintain agency over your health ecosystem even when certain aspects of your physical function are permanently altered.

11

When Disability Informs the Ecosystem

Patients often struggle to make the connection between declining phys-ical function and worsening health. A person who has stopped cooking due to nerve pain or weakness may not report this during a doctor's visit, instead describing symptoms of fatigue or poor appetite without linking them to the inability to prepare proper meals. Someone with a permanent disability may not mention their daily pain medication routine for fear of being judged or misunderstood—or because they have become accustomed to their physical limitation. Others may be reluctant to admit that they need help, worrying about losing their independence or assuming that there's nothing else to be done.

This disconnect means that physical struggles are often an invisible source of medical problems, one that requires active, probing questioning by healthcare providers to uncover. It also requires skeletal awareness and self-advocacy on the patient's side. This chapter explores what happens when your physical infrastructure—your ability to move through the world—faces more permanent challenges.

The Hidden Epidemic of Physical Limitation

Physical disabilities are more common than many people realize, affecting an estimated 16 percent of the global population and nearly 25 percent of adults in the United States. These disabilities range from mobility impairments due to arthritis, stroke, or neurological conditions to chronic pain and musculoskeletal disorders that limit movement. While disability itself is not a disease, it often intersects with health in ways that create additional challenges. People with limited mobility are at higher risk for secondary health issues, including cardiovascular disease, osteoporosis, pressure ulcers, and depression. Many of these complications arise not directly from the disability itself but from barriers to movement, inadequate access to healthcare, and the social isolation that often accompanies physical impairments.

Despite the prevalence of disability, medical care is often focused on treating individual symptoms—high blood pressure, recurrent infections, or malnutrition—without recognizing how an underlying loss of physical function might be driving these issues. Difficulties in performing activities of daily living (ADLs) can be an overlooked driver of health, often masquerading as purely medical problems. The Katz Index of Independence in Activities of Daily Living includes questions such as: Can you bathe yourself without assistance? Do you need help getting dressed? Can you use the toilet independently? Are you able to prepare your own meals? Physicians, caregivers, and even patients themselves often fail to recognize difficulties with activities of daily living as the root cause of medical problems.

A person who struggles to bathe, dress, or prepare meals due to arthritis or frailty may develop recurrent infections, unintended weight loss, or worsening diabetes—not because of the disease process but because they physically can't complete tasks essential to their well-being. Similarly, someone who has trouble walking may avoid necessary medical visits, leading to missed diagnoses or untreated conditions. In a rushed clinical setting, doctors may focus on treating measurable symptoms—uncontrolled blood sugar, frequent falls, malnutrition—without digging deeper into whether a patient's functional limitations are driving these issues. When these functional limitations go unaddressed, patients may be prescribed additional medications or treatments without tackling the root cause: their inability to care for themselves independently.

A physician might prescribe stronger diabetes medication for a patient whose blood sugar is erratic without realizing that vision problems or arthritis prevent them from reliably administering insulin. Similarly, a patient with frequent urinary tract infections may be prescribed multiple rounds of antibiotics, when the real issue is difficulty with personal hygiene due to mobility challenges. Without explicitly assessing a person's ability to manage basic tasks, well-intentioned medical professionals can overlook the most effective solutions: home health support, physical therapy, or assistive devices that enable a person to live more safely and independently.

That disconnect was a key issue for Marion, a vibrant sixty-seven-year-old former high school principal who received a Parkinson's diagnosis five years ago. The disease had gradually affected her balance and gait, giving her a characteristic shuffling walk. She had already experienced two falls at home, fortunately without serious injury. When I first met Marion, she mentioned feeling dizzy when standing up quickly. Her blood pressure readings in my office were consistently low at 102/68 mmHg. A review of her medication list revealed that she was taking both a beta-blocker for her heart and her Parkinson's medications, a combination that was likely contributing to her orthostatic hypotension, the sudden drop in blood pressure when she stood up.

"I'm so worried about falling," she confessed during our appointment. "My friend broke her hip last year, and she never really recovered. I've started avoiding going out unless someone's with me."

Her fear wasn't irrational. For older adults, falls are a serious health risk that can trigger a cascade of complications. But Marion's situation highlighted a common challenge in managing complex health conditions: Sometimes treating one problem creates vulnerability in another area. We needed to think about her health as interconnected systems—specifically the effects of Parkinson's disease on her balance, her medications on her blood pressure, and her blood pressure on her fall risk. Rather than treating each issue separately, we needed to look at the bigger picture. After consulting with her neurologist and cardiologist, we made a decision to reduce her blood pressure medication, allowing her blood pressure readings to float higher than ideal targets. That would reduce her risk of dizziness when standing up, which was compounding her balance difficulties due to Parkinson's.

"But I thought lower blood pressure was always better," Marion commented.

"In your case," I explained, "the risk of falls due to low blood pressure may outweigh the risk of slightly higher readings." Optimizing each number in isolation wasn't the goal (it also wasn't possible); the goal was finding the right balance for her overall health. We complemented that approach with physical therapy focused specifically on balance training and fall prevention. Marion's therapist taught her strategies for safer movement: how to turn her entire body rather than just her head, how to rise from sitting without triggering dizziness, and exercises to strengthen her core and leg muscles.

Six months later, Marion reported having had no falls despite her Parkinson's progression. Her blood pressure readings had settled around 130/80 mmHg, higher than before but still within a reasonable range. More important, she'd regained confidence in her ability to move through the world, resuming her weekly bridge games and even joining a seated tai chi class designed for people with movement disorders.

Marion's case illustrates a crucial principle in managing health with chronic conditions: Sometimes we need to accept strategic trade-offs. By allowing her blood pressure to run higher than what might be ideal in other circumstances, we reduced her overall risk profile. Her health wasn't defined by a single number but by her functioning, safety, and quality of life.

Disability's Impact on Your Other Health Quadrants

When disability affects your INFRASTRUCTURE quadrant, it inevitably creates ripple effects throughout your INFORMATICS and INPUTS quadrants as well. Understanding these relationships can help you develop more effective coping strategies and maintain greater agency over your health.

Physical limitations often change your medical data, sometimes in ways that require careful interpretation. For instance, someone unable to walk regularly due to chronic pain might show higher cholesterol levels or blood pressure readings than they would if fully mobile. While these readings can't be ignored, they may need to be understood in context rather than just compared to standard benchmarks. Similarly, traditional assessment tools may not capture the full picture for those with disabilities. Standard depression questionnaires, for example, often include physical symptoms that might be present due to disability rather than mood disorder. This can lead to overdiagnosis or inappropriate treatment if not carefully considered.

The relationship works both ways: Medical data can also help guide adaptations to disability. Regular monitoring of vitals and lab values can reveal when practical workarounds for physical limitations are effective and when they need adjustment. For example, a person with limited arm mobility might develop a technique for self-administering medication using adaptive equipment. Blood tests showing consistent medication levels would confirm that this approach is working, while erratic results might indicate that the technique needs refinement. This data shouldn't dictate life choices but can provide useful feedback for fine-tuning approaches to maintaining independence despite physical limitations.

Physical limitations can significantly impact what you eat, drink, and otherwise consume. Someone with limited hand dexterity might struggle to prepare nutritious meals, leading to greater reliance on processed, easy-to-prepare foods. A person with swallowing difficulties may face challenges getting adequate hydration or nutrition. Mobility impairments can make grocery shopping difficult, limiting access to fresh foods. Certain disabilities also affect how the body processes medications, supplements, and other substances. For example, reduced physical activity can alter drug metabolism, potentially requiring dosage adjustments. Gastrointestinal issues that accompany some disabilities might affect nutrient absorption, creating a need for specific supplementation.

Conversely, what you consume can profoundly affect how you experience disability. Proper hydration can reduce the muscle cramping of many neuromuscular conditions. Anti-inflammatory foods may help manage pain in arthritic conditions. Sleep-promoting habits can enhance energy reserves for those with limited stamina. These interconnections underscore the importance of considering your full health ecosystem when adapting to disability. No single intervention—whether medical, nutritional, or physical—exists in isolation. The most effective approaches integrate all of them.

When Pain Becomes the Center of Existence

Chronic pain is perhaps one of the most profoundly misunderstood phenomena in medicine, simultaneously ubiquitous and invisible. Affecting an estimated 50 million Americans, chronic pain isn't merely a symptom but a complex neurobiological condition that can become the central organizing force in a patient's health. When pain persists beyond three to six months, it fundamentally rewires the nervous system, creating a cascade of physiological changes that extend far beyond the initial injury or illness. The body enters a state of constant stress response, triggering inflammation, hormonal disruptions, and neurochemical imbalances that affect virtually every bodily system. Yet in the fragmented landscape of modern healthcare, this all-encompassing influence often goes unrecognized.

Ray's story exemplifies how chronic pain can become the central driver of a person's entire health ecosystem. At fifty-two, a serious construction accident had left him with a crushed vertebra and persistent back pain that had never subsided despite several surgeries. When he came to see me, his medical chart was thick with diagnoses—hypertension, prediabetes, depression, gastric issues—and a list of medications that required its own page in his electronic record. He had seen at least eight specialists in three years: neurologist, orthopedist, gastroenterologist, endocrinologist, cardiologist, psychiatrist, pain specialist, and sleep doctor. Each had approached their piece of the puzzle in isolation. "I need something stronger for the pain, Doc," Ray said during our appointment. "The hydrocodone barely takes the edge off anymore."

As we talked about his daily life, a pattern emerged. His inability to exercise due to pain had contributed to his weight gain, which had worsened his back problems and led to prediabetes. Poor sleep from pain fed his depression. The pain medications caused gastric problems requiring acid reducers. The NSAIDs he took strained his liver. "Ray, your pain isn't just a symptom; it's become the center of a wheel, with all these other health issues radiating out from it like spokes," I explained. "Each specialist has been treating individual spokes, but we haven't effectively addressed the hub."

This pattern is common in modern medicine. Medical training traditionally frames pain as a warning signal—a symptom pointing to an underlying problem that, once resolved, should eliminate the pain. This paradigm works beautifully for acute conditions but fails catastrophically when applied to chronic pain. Physicians, trained to think in terms of discrete diagnoses and targeted treatments, may continue hunting for structural abnormalities long after pain has evolved into a self-perpetuating neurological condition. In Ray's case, rather than simply increasing his pain medication again, we developed a comprehensive approach: a pain rehabilitation program that included physical therapy designed for chronic pain patients, cognitive behavioral therapy to address the psychological dimensions of his pain, a gradual increase in activity to rebuild strength, and medication optimization that actually meant reducing some prescriptions rather than adding more.

Six months into the program, Ray's transformation was remarkable. His pain hadn't disappeared completely, but his functional capacity had improved significantly. He could cook dinner with his wife and had begun taking short walks. His blood pressure had stabilized, his blood sugar levels had improved, and we'd eliminated three of his medications. He still had pain, but the pain didn't own him. The crucial insight in his case was recognizing that his chronic pain wasn't just a symptom to be medicated but a condition that had reshaped his entire health landscape. By addressing how pain had restructured his life rather than simply trying to eliminate it, we helped him reclaim function and meaning.

Finding the Middle Path: The Balance Between Acceptance and Agency

What connects Marion's and Ray's stories are not just their physical challenges but how those challenges transformed their entire health ecosystems. In each case, their conditions couldn't be fully "fixed" in the traditional medical sense. Instead, they needed approaches that acknowledged their physical limitations while finding new paths to agency. These examples highlight a fundamental truth: Disability doesn't happen in isolation. Physical limitations create ripple effects throughout our health, requiring us to make thoughtful trade-offs and redefine what well-being means within new constraints.

For Marion, that meant accepting that her Parkinson's would progress but finding ways to maintain safety despite it. For Ray, it meant shifting the focus from simply eliminating pain to rebuilding function alongside it. Breaking the cycle of symptom-focused treatment requires a paradigm shift—recognizing that conditions such as chronic pain and physical disability are not merely symptoms but complex conditions that drive numerous physical and psychological changes throughout the body. When physicians widen their lenses to see how these conditions affect sleep, mood, activity levels, stress hormones, and immune function, they can begin to address the full spectrum of health issues with integrated approaches rather than fragmented symptom management.

Practical Strategies for Navigating Disability

If you're facing a new diagnosis or progression of a chronic condition that affects your physical function, consider these approaches:

- **Assemble your team.** Beyond medical specialists, consider physical and occupational therapists, mental health professionals, nutritionists, and social workers who can help address the full spectrum of your needs.
- **Adapt your environment before crisis hits.** Simple modifications—grab bars, shower seats, elevated toilet seats, kitchen adaptations—can prevent injuries and maintain independence. Don't wait until after a fall or other crisis occurs to make these changes.
- **Prioritize energy conservation.** If you have limited physical reserves, be strategic about how you spend them. Focus on activities that bring meaning and joy rather than exhausting yourself with tasks that could be delegated or adapted.
- **Lean into assistive technology.** From mobility aids to medication dispensers to smart home features, technology can bridge gaps created by physical limitations.
- **Build community.** Connect with others who understand your experiences through support groups, online communities, or adaptive activity programs. Shared wisdom can provide both practical solutions and emotional support.
- **Practice acceptance—actively.** Acceptance isn't passive resignation but an active practice of acknowledging reality while still seeking agency within it. Mindfulness practices can help cultivate this balance.
- **Reassess regularly.** As conditions progress or change, solutions that worked before may need adjustment. Regular check-ins with healthcare providers and honest self-assessment can help keep your approach aligned with your current needs.

No one navigates disability entirely alone. A crucial part of maintaining health with physical limitations is building the right support system: healthcare providers who understand your specific needs, friends and family who provide practical and emotional support, and sometimes professional caregivers who provide specialized assistance.

Having to rely on such a support system isn't a sign of weakness or dependence. Rather, it's a strategic deployment of resources that allows you to direct your limited energy toward what matters most. Just as a CEO delegates certain tasks to others in order to focus on strategic priorities, someone living with disability must sometimes delegate aspects of daily function to preserve energy for what brings meaning and joy. A more holistic approach—one that considers physical ability, home environment, and social support—can help reframe disability-related issues and provide targeted interventions from physical therapy to in-home care that will improve both independence and overall health outcomes.

Technology and Adaptation: Modern Tools for Independence

The intersection of disability and technology has created unprecedented opportunities for maintaining independence and health management. Modern assistive technology extends far beyond traditional mobility aids—today's tools include voice-activated home systems, adaptive gaming controllers that enable people with limited hand function to continue hobbies they love, and health monitoring devices that help people with chronic conditions identify patterns and manage their care. My patient Ralph, who has progressive multiple sclerosis, exemplifies this strategic approach: As his hand dexterity declined, simple tools like automatic pill dispensers and ergonomic kitchen utensils (most under $50) allowed him to maintain control over his daily medication routine and continue cooking. "It's not about the money," he told me. "It's about still being able to take care of myself in ways that matter to me."

The key is matching technology to your specific needs rather than chasing what's newest or most sophisticated. Before investing, identify your functional challenges, consider your comfort level with technology, and start simple. Occupational therapists who specialize in assistive technology can help navigate options. Technology shouldn't replace human connection, but it can facilitate it—video calling enables face-to-face communication when travel is difficult, and online communities connect people with similar conditions for support and shared wisdom.

The goal isn't to accumulate gadgets but to thoughtfully employ technology that improves your daily life. The best assistive technology becomes invisible, seamlessly enabling you to focus on what matters most rather than drawing attention to limitations.

Mindfulness and Movement: Tools for Adaptation

For many people with chronic conditions or disabilities, mindfulness practices offer powerful tools for navigating their changed relationship with their bodies. Unlike the harmful messaging that suggests that you can overcome any physical limitation through sheer willpower, mindfulness approaches encourage you to work with your body rather than against it. Practices such as adaptive yoga, tai chi, and meditation help develop awareness of what your body needs in each moment. They teach you to notice when you're pushing too hard and when you have capacity for more. They help you become attuned to subtle signals that might indicate an impending flare-up or the need for rest.

Movement itself becomes medicine—not the intense exercise that might be impossible with certain limitations but gentle, intentional movement that helps maintain function and reduce pain. For someone with severe arthritis, this might mean range-of-motion exercises in warm water. For someone with Parkinson's, it might mean specialized boxing classes that improve coordination and balance. What matters isn't the specific practice but the principle: working with your body's current capabilities rather than fighting against its limitations or ignoring its signals. This mindful approach fosters a compassionate relationship with your changed physical reality, reducing the emotional suffering that often accompanies physical limitations.

The Paradox of Limitation

There is a paradox at the heart of disability: Physical limitations can simultaneously restrict certain freedoms while opening unexpected doors to new perspectives, deeper connections, and more authentic engagement with life. The most profound wisdom often comes from those who have navigated significant constraints. This doesn't romanticize or minimize the very real difficulties of physical disability. Pain is still pain. Limitation is still limitation. Loss deserves to be acknowledged and grieved. But within that honest acknowledgment lies the possibility of transformation—of finding new ways to engage with the world, with others, and with yourself.

Too often, society equates health with perfect physical function and complete independence, while those living with disabilities are framed as inherently "unhealthy" regardless of their actual well-being. But what if we were to expand our definition? What if health isn't about the absence of disease or limitation but about creating meaning, connection, and joy within whatever physical reality we inhabit? What if it's not about comparing ourselves to an idealized physical standard but about developing our unique capacities within our particular circumstances?

This redefinition isn't just relevant for those with disabilities; it offers wisdom for anyone navigating the physical changes that come with age. None of us will maintain perfect physical function throughout our lives. All of us will eventually face some form of limitation. The question isn't whether this will happen but how we'll respond when it does. The body you have may not be the one you expected or hoped for. It may have capabilities and limitations different from others'. But it remains the vehicle that carries you through this life, worthy of care, adaptation, and profound respect for all it continues to make possible.

The balancing act between acceptance of our limitations and agency over the areas we can control represents the middle path: neither surrendering to injury nor denying the reality of disability but finding a way forward that honors what we've lost and what remains possible.

KNOW YOURSELF, ADVOCATE FOR YOURSELF
Your INFRASTRUCTURE Reflection and Action Guide

PART 1 Self-Reflection: Understanding Your INFRASTRUCTURE Quadrant

Grab your pen and paper or laptop again. Now we'll explore your physical container, the "house" that carries your entire health ecosystem.

Your Body's Current State

- When you wake up in the morning, what hurts? What feels strong?
- Think about your typical day—what physical tasks do you avoid or modify because of how your body feels?
- How has your body's capability changed in the past five years? Ten years?
- What types of movement make you feel good—energized, capable, alive?
- What movements make you anxious, uncomfortable, or remind you of limitations?
- Does your home, workplace, or community make it easy or hard to move the way you'd like to?
- Have you developed workarounds for physical limitations—like always using one arm to carry things, or avoiding stairs, or sitting in certain positions?

Your Relationship with Your Body

- How good are you at noticing when something feels "off" in your body before it becomes a real problem?
- Can you tell the difference between "good pain" (like sore muscles after exercise) and "bad pain" (like injury)?
- How do you feel about your body's capabilities right now? Grateful? Frustrated? Accepting?
- Have past injuries or physical challenges changed how you think about your body?

Connections Across Your Health

- Does physical discomfort or fatigue affect what or when you eat, drink, or consume?

- How does what you put into your body affect your physical container (like sugar or gluten causing joint pains)?
- How do your aches, pains, or physical limitations show up in your medical data (like elevated blood pressure when you're in pain or high cholesterol when you can't exercise regularly)?

Reclaiming Agency

- Where do you feel you have real control over your physical container?
- Where do you feel powerless or stuck?
- What's one realistic change you could make that would improve how your body feels or functions (like stretching or engaging in physical therapy)?
- What's one realistic change you could make in your physical activity that would improve your medical data (like weight-lifting to improve bone density or cardiovascular exercise to reduce blood sugar readings)?

PART 2 Healthcare Conversations: Questions and Strategies for Medical Encounters

Questions to Ask Your Doctor

- "How might my [past injuries/skeletal complaints/activity/movement pattern] be contributing to my symptoms?"
- "What types of movement would be most beneficial for my specific condition?"
- "Are there any evidence-based physical therapy approaches for this type of pain/limitation?"
- "How can I safely maintain activity while managing this condition?"
- "How can I distinguish between challenging my body and potentially injuring it?"
- "What warning signs should I watch for that would indicate that I need to modify my activity?"
- "Are there specialists I should see for my physical concerns, and if so, when?"
- "What adaptive equipment or modifications might help me maintain my independence?"

Communication Strategies

- Bring a list of all past injuries and accidents and all skeletal surgeries, known asymmetries, and limitations.
- Demonstrate exactly how and where you experience pain/discomfort.
- Ask for referrals to movement specialists when appropriate.
- Ask if it's more appropriate to see a physical therapist or an orthopedist for your condition and why.
- Request written instructions for recommended exercises.
- Discuss how to modify activities you enjoy rather than eliminating them.
- Be honest about your current activity level and any barriers you face.
- Ask for specific guidance on when to seek urgent care for physical symptoms.

Consider keeping notes on these reflections to reference as we continue to build your complete health ecosystem in the remaining quadrant.

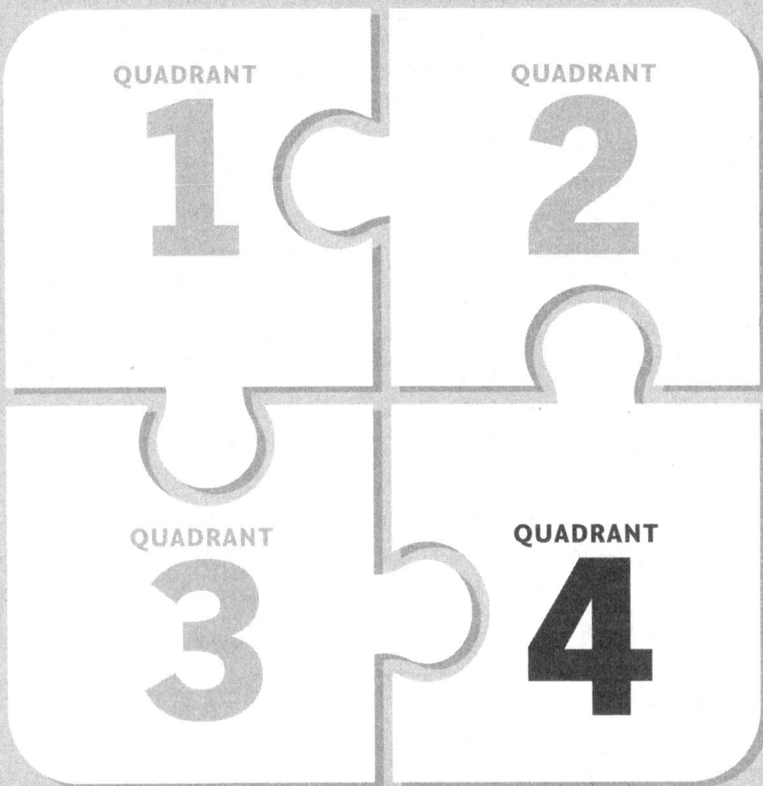

INSIGHT

You've arrived at the INSIGHT quadrant. It encompasses a vast internal territory from your conscious mental healthcare to the hidden cognitive biases that shape your daily choices. This may be the most powerful quadrant of all.

Your mental state directly influences every number in your INFORMATICS quadrant: Chronic stress elevates cortisol and blood sugar, depression suppresses immune function, and anxiety can spike blood pressure. It drives your INPUTS quadrant: emotional eating, stress drinking, and the supplements you buy when wellness anxiety peaks. It shapes your INFRASTRUCTURE quadrant: When you're depressed, exercise feels impossible; when you're anxious, your muscles carry tension that creates pain.

Yet for too long, mental health has been treated as the stepchild of "real" medicine—an optional add-on rather than the foundation it is. Everyone has mental health, just as everyone has cardiovascular health or immune health. It exists on a continuum that we all move along throughout our lives. Some of us have a genetic predisposition to anxiety or mood disorders, but no one escapes stress, grief, relationship challenges, and the cognitive changes that come with aging. Mental health isn't about being "crazy" or "normal"; it's about understanding how your mind works and caring for it with intention.

Your INSIGHT quadrant includes both the obvious and the hidden. It encompasses the optimism that propels you forward in life and the perfectionism you don't recognize as anxiety. It includes your conscious fears about mortality and your unconscious feelings of self-doubt. It covers your sharp memory and periodic brain fog, as well as the stories you tell yourself about your body, your worth, and your future.

Understanding your INSIGHT means recognizing that mental health is health, that your thoughts have biological consequences, and that the most sustainable health changes often begin not with your diet or exercise routine, but with your relationship to yourself. It means seeing that the voice in your head—critical or compassionate, fearful or curious—shapes every health decision you make.

By the end of this section, you'll understand how to befriend your mind rather than fight it, how to recognize when you need support, and how to harness the most powerful tool in your health arsenal: your own awareness.

12

Mental Health Is Health

The relationship between your mental health and your physical health is deeply intertwined. When you experience chronic anxiety, your body responds with a cascade of stress hormones that, over time, can contribute to hypertension, cardiovascular disease, and immune dysfunction. Depression symptoms not only affect your mood, they change your eating patterns, sleep architecture, and inflammation levels. Studies consistently show that mental health conditions increase the risk of developing chronic diseases, while also making those diseases harder to manage.

Conversely, physical illness often precipitates mental health challenges. Consider the patient who develops depression following a cancer diagnosis or anxiety after a heart attack. Chronic pain frequently coexists with mood disorders, creating a vicious cycle in which each condition amplifies the other. Even conditions such as diabetes can affect brain function through blood sugar fluctuations, impacting cognitive performance and emotional regulation.

Our healthcare system often treats these connections as incidental rather than fundamental. We medicate depression without referencing the underlying physical shifts that triggered it. We prescribe pain medication without exploring how trauma might be manifesting as physical discomfort. This siloed approach not only fails to address root causes but often creates new problems due to interactions among pharmaceuticals as well as missed opportunities for healing.

The most compelling evidence for the mind-body interconnection comes from interventions that target both domains simultaneously. Exercise, for example, improves both depression and cardiovascular health. Mindfulness practices reduce anxiety while lowering blood pressure. By acknowledging these connections rather than treating mind and body as separate entities, we open new pathways to healing and wellness.

But mental health is not merely the absence of diagnosable psychiatric conditions. It's not a binary state of "well" versus "ill" but a dynamic continuum that we all move along throughout our lives. At its core, mental health encompasses your emotional, psychological, and social well-being—how you think, feel, and relate to yourself and others.

Despite what wellness influencers might suggest, mental health doesn't mean feeling perpetually positive or completely eliminating uncomfortable emotions. Anxiety, sadness, anger, and grief are normal, necessary aspects of the human experience, not pathologies to be eradicated. The goal isn't to never feel these emotions but to develop a relationship with them that doesn't impair functioning or cause excessive suffering.

Sometimes the pursuit of constant happiness becomes a source of distress itself. Patients tell me that they feel guilty or broken for experiencing natural emotional responses to difficult circumstances. This "happiness imperative" can paradoxically worsen mental health by creating unrealistic expectations and self-judgment.

Healthy minds experience the full spectrum of human emotion. They're resilient rather than impervious—able to feel deeply, process emotions effectively, and return to baseline rather than becoming stuck in maladaptive patterns. This emotional flexibility, not the absence of negative feelings, is the hallmark of robust mental health.

Mental health challenges affect people across all demographic lines, from the CEO to the service worker, from the suburban family to the urban single, from those living in a religious community to those inhabiting secular spaces. While poverty and marginalization create stressors that increase vulnerability, no amount of privilege provides immunity from depression, anxiety, or other mental health conditions.

I've treated wealthy executives whose anxiety made their success feel meaningless and working-class patients whose resilience in the face of multiple adversities was nothing short of remarkable. Material comfort can provide resources for addressing mental health issues but doesn't prevent them from developing. Conversely, economic hardship creates barriers to care but doesn't define one's capacity to achieve emotional well-being.

This recognition can help you move beyond the harmful narrative that mental health problems reflect some failure of lifestyle optimization. The notion that one can simply "habit stack" their way out of clinical depression or severe anxiety disorder reflects a fundamental misunderstanding of these conditions. While consistent sleep, regular exercise, and mindfulness practices undoubtedly contribute to mental well-being, they're rarely sufficient alone for addressing significant mental health challenges.

You can meditate daily, exercise regularly, eat a "perfect" diet, and maintain an immaculate work-life balance and still develop depression. You can live with significant material constraints and still cultivate meaningful emotional resilience. Mental health isn't a luxury good or a lifestyle achievement; it's a fundamental part of the human experience. Similarly, mental health isn't simply a matter of disciplined habits, though routine and structure can certainly support it. While substance use can certainly complicate mental health, abstinence alone doesn't guarantee emotional well-being. I've seen patients maintain perfect sobriety while still struggling with the underlying anxiety or trauma that initially drove their substance use. Conversely, I've worked with patients who occasionally use substances in moderation while maintaining robust mental health through other supportive practices.

This isn't to minimize the importance of behavioral choices in supporting mental health but rather to challenge the narrative that mental illness reflects some failure of willpower or personal discipline. Such framing often compounds suffering by adding shame to an already difficult experience.

Perfect performance as a parent, spouse, or worker also doesn't define mental health, nor does struggling in these domains necessarily indicate poor mental health. Parents with anxiety can raise securely attached children. Professionals with depression can make valuable contributions in the workplace. Caregivers with their own health challenges can provide compassionate support to others.

The perfectionism that often drives our expectations can itself become a liability. Setting impossible standards and then judging oneself harshly for inevitable shortfalls creates a breeding ground for anxiety and depression. Many patients come to me not because they're failing at life but because they're exhausting themselves trying to achieve perfection in multiple domains simultaneously.

Healthy mental functioning allows for balance, boundaries, and self-compassion. It means recognizing our limitations, prioritizing what matters most, and allowing ourselves to be human in our various roles. Sometimes the most healing step is releasing the expectation of being an exceptional performer in every area of life and embracing the reality of being "good enough."

Mental Health as a Process

Just as physical health requires ongoing maintenance, mental health "upkeep" is a continual process, too. This process begins with cultivating self-awareness: recognizing your patterns, triggers, and emotional responses without judgment. It progresses through acceptance of both your struggles and your strengths, your fixed vulnerabilities and your capacity for growth. From this foundation of awareness and acceptance emerges genuine agency—the ability to make conscious choices about your thoughts, feelings, and behaviors rather than being driven by unconscious patterns.

This process isn't linear; all of us cycle through stages repeatedly as we encounter new challenges and life phases. The college student who developed effective anxiety management strategies may need to revisit these practices during the transition to parenthood. The executive who's maintained a stable mood for years through medication and therapy might require additional support during a period of grief or career transition.

Mental health as a process embraces the full human experience, including the painful, difficult, and messy aspects and events that are inevitable in every life. Rather than chasing the illusion of perfect mental health, I recommend engaging with your inner landscape to foster resilience, meaning, and a sturdy sense of self.

How Mental Health Conditions Affect Your Health Ecosystem

Mental health conditions don't just affect your mood or thoughts; they create ripple effects throughout your entire health ecosystem. Understanding these connections is crucial to developing truly effective approaches to well-being.

Mental Health and the INFORMATICS Quadrant

Mental health challenges often appear in medical data in subtle ways: as elevated inflammation markers, disrupted sleep patterns on fitness trackers, or blood pressure changes during stressful periods. Understanding these connections, which we explored in the INFORMATICS quadrant, helps both patients and providers recognize the full scope of mental health's impact. Consider how anxiety and depression affect your physiological measurements:

- **Blood pressure and heart rate:** Anxiety disorders can elevate blood pressure and heart rate, potentially leading to misdiagnosis of primary hypertension when the underlying issue is psychological distress. I've had patients whose medication dosages were repeatedly increased when what they really needed was treatment for anxiety.

- **Inflammatory markers:** Depression and chronic stress increase inflammatory markers such as C-reactive protein and interleukin-6, which are associated with increased risk of developing cardiovascular disease, diabetes, and other chronic conditions. These elevations aren't just correlations; they represent direct biological pathways through which mental health affects physical health outcomes.
- **Blood sugar regulation:** Anxiety triggers cortisol release, which elevates the blood glucose level. For patients with diabetes or prediabetes, psychological distress can make glucose control significantly more challenging, creating frustrating patterns that don't respond to standard diabetes management approaches.
- **Pain perception:** Depression and anxiety lower pain thresholds and amplify pain signals, creating situations in which standard pain assessments may not capture the complex interplay between emotional distress and physical sensations. This helps explain why patients with these conditions often experience pain more intensely and require different management approaches.
- **Cognitive health:** The relationship between mental and physical health extends to cognitive function as well. Chronic anxiety doesn't just affect mood; it can also impair memory consolidation and attention control. Depression influences not only emotional regulation but also processing speed and executive function. As we'll explore in chapter 13, understanding these cognitive dimensions of mental health helps us develop more comprehensive approaches to brain care.
- **Medication metabolism:** Your mental health can even affect how your body processes medications. Depression alters liver enzyme activity, potentially changing how quickly your body metabolizes certain drugs and affecting optimal dosing. This is another example of how mental health conditions aren't just "comorbidities" but fundamental influences on your entire health picture.

Chris, a forty-two-year-old biotech professional, came to me convinced that he had a progressive neurological disease such as multiple sclerosis or amyotrophic lateral sclerosis (ALS). He fixated on minor symptoms such as an eye twitch and occasional toe numbness and spent hours researching rare conditions online. Meanwhile, his actual health data revealed concerning but less dramatic issues: prediabetes, elevated cholesterol, and abnormal liver function likely related to his weekend alcohol use. His anxiety about his health wasn't just an emotional issue; it was creating measurable health consequences by diverting his attention from addressable risk factors while simultaneously elevating his stress hormones through constant worry.

When we addressed his underlying anxiety with therapy and mindfulness techniques, not only did his neurological fears subside, but his metabolic markers improved as well. His blood pressure normalized, his liver enzymes decreased, and he became motivated to address his prediabetes through lifestyle changes. This case illustrates how mental health interventions can improve "physical" health metrics by addressing the interconnected nature of our health ecosystem.

Mental Health and the INPUTS Quadrant

"What's eating you?" This common phrase denotes the obvious, inextricable relationship between what we consume and how we feel. The caffeine that provides morning alertness can worsen anxiety symptoms (as discussed in the INPUTS quadrant). The alcohol used to manage stress can disrupt sleep and ultimately exacerbate mood disorders. There are several ways that our INPUTS can impact our INSIGHT.

- **Emotional eating:** Mood disorders frequently drive problematic eating patterns, whether restricting food during depression, binge eating to soothe anxiety, or using sugar for temporary mood enhancement. These behaviors aren't just psychological; they create physiological consequences that further affect mood, creating challenging cycles.

- **Self-medication:** Many patients use alcohol, cannabis, or other substances to manage anxiety or depression symptoms. While this may provide temporary relief, it often exacerbates the underlying condition through rebound anxiety, disrupted sleep architecture, or neurochemical changes that intensify depressive symptoms.
- **Medication compliance:** Mental health conditions can significantly impact whether patients take prescribed medications as directed. Depression may cause them to forget doses or feel too hopeless to bother, while anxiety might lead to either avoidance of medications due to fear of side effects or overuse of as-needed medications such as benzodiazepines.
- **Nutritional impact:** Some mental health conditions create nutritional challenges that affect the entire body. Restrictive eating patterns in anxiety disorders may lead to deficiencies in B vitamins, omega-3 fatty acids, and other nutrients crucial for neurological function, potentially worsening the very symptoms they're trying to manage.

Brett, a forty-five-year-old endurance athlete, came to me with severe low-back pain from a herniated disc and growing frustration about his inability to maintain his training schedule. As we explored his history, I discovered that since adolescence, he had used intense exercise to manage his undiagnosed ADHD. Exercise provided the dopamine his brain craved, helping him focus and feel regulated. When injury prevented his usual training, he experienced not just physical pain but a neurochemical deficit that manifested itself as irritability, difficulty concentrating, and growing anxiety. His attempts to push through the pain were creating a cycle of injury and inadequate healing. This wasn't just about athletic determination; it was his unconscious attempt to self-medicate a neurological condition through physical activity.

By addressing his ADHD with appropriate treatment, Brett found a better balance in his approach to recovery, allowing proper healing while supporting his brain's need for dopamine regulation. This case highlights how mental health conditions often drive input choices in ways that significantly impact physical health, creating cycles that can't be broken by addressing just one dimension.

Mental health's impact extends beyond what you consume to how you move your body. Let's explore these dynamics within our INFRASTRUCTURE quadrant.

Mental Health and the INFRASTRUCTURE Quadrant

Physical movement serves as both symptom management and prevention for mental health challenges. The exercise discussed in the INFRASTRUCTURE quadrant directly influences neurotransmitter production, stress hormone regulation, and mood stability—demonstrating the profound connection between body and mind.

- **Muscle tension patterns:** Anxiety disorders create characteristic muscle tension patterns that can lead to pain, postural changes, and movement compensations. A person with chronic anxiety often develops upper trapezius muscle tightness, forward head posture, and shallow breathing patterns that compound their physical discomfort.
- **Avoidance of movement:** Depression frequently leads to decreased physical activity, which creates a cascade of physiological consequences: muscle atrophy, decreased cardiovascular capacity, compromised immune function, and worsening mood through reduced endorphin release. This self-reinforcing cycle can be difficult to interrupt without addressing the mental and physical components simultaneously.
- **Body awareness:** Many mental health conditions involve some degree of disconnection from bodily sensations—either a hyperfocus on certain sensations (as in health anxiety) or a diminished awareness of physical needs (as in depression). This altered body awareness can lead to movement patterns that create or exacerbate physical problems.

- **Sleep position and quality:** Mental health significantly affects sleep posture and quality, which directly impacts musculoskeletal health. Anxiety may cause restless sleep with frequent position changes that prevent tissue recovery, while depression might result in prolonged immobility in poor positions that strain joints and soft tissues.

Michael, a forty-five-year-old software engineer struggling with obsessive-compulsive disorder (OCD), presented with irritable bowel syndrome (IBS) that hadn't responded to conventional treatments. Closer examination revealed that his compulsive behaviors included excessive abdominal muscle tensing throughout the day, an unconscious attempt to feel "in control" that was disrupting his normal gut motility.

His mental health condition wasn't just affecting his thoughts; it was literally changing his physical structure and function. By addressing the OCD through appropriate therapy and medication while simultaneously working with a physical therapist on diaphragmatic breathing and abdominal relaxation, we created an integrated approach that addressed both his mental patterns and their physical manifestations. His IBS symptoms improved dramatically not because we found the right digestive medication but because we recognized the mind-body connection driving his symptoms.

The Inseparability of Social-Emotional, Behavioral, and Mental Health

Mental health is directly tied to social context, behavior, and emotional factors. Loneliness and social isolation have emerged as public health crises, with research showing that their impact on mortality is comparable to that of smoking or obesity. Workplace stress, financial insecurity, and relationship dysfunction all create fertile ground for anxiety and depression to take root. Even our digital habits—constant connectivity, social media comparison, and sleep disruption due to screen use—shape our mental landscape in ways we're only beginning to understand.

As we discussed in the INFORMATICS chapter on biographic data, these social-emotional factors don't just correlate with mental health challenges; they can directly cause them. A child growing up with chronic stress develops different neural pathways from one who is raised in stability. An adult experiencing workplace bullying may develop anxiety that persists long after changing jobs. Someone lacking meaningful social connection is at substantially higher risk for depression.

The reverse is equally true: Mental health conditions profoundly affect our social functioning and behavioral choices. Depression leads to withdrawal from relationships. Anxiety creates avoidance patterns that limit life opportunities. Substance use disorders disrupt family systems and workplace performance. These behavioral manifestations often trigger judgment rather than compassion, creating stigma that further isolates those suffering and prevents them from seeking help.

In each case, focusing solely on symptom management without addressing the person's broader emotional ecosystem is like treating a fish's illness without examining the water it swims in. Healing requires acknowledging the complex interplay between our internal and external worlds.

The Neurobiology of Emotions

Emotions aren't abstract concepts that exist only in the mind; they have measurable physiological signatures. Fear quickens our heart rate, constricts our breathing, and diverts blood flow from our digestive system to our muscles. Joy releases dopamine and endorphins that reduce pain perception. Chronic grief alters immune function. This isn't metaphorical; it's biological.

The vagus nerve forms a direct superhighway between brain and body, transmitting emotional states throughout your internal organs. Your gut contains its own nervous system (the enteric nervous system), which has more neurons than your spinal cord and communicates constantly with your brain. Your immune system, once thought to operate independently, is now known to be deeply influenced by your psychological state.

These connections help explain phenomena that conventional medicine struggles to address. Why does stress trigger IBS flares? Why do trauma survivors experience higher rates of autoimmune conditions? Why do some patients with anxiety report physical symptoms—racing heart, shortness of breath, gastrointestinal distress—more prominently than emotional ones?

I've seen countless patients who've cycled through specialists seeking explanations for physical symptoms that ultimately stemmed from their unaddressed emotional health issues. Conversely, I've treated patients whose psychiatric symptoms improved dramatically when their underlying physical conditions were properly addressed. This isn't to suggest that their symptoms were "all in their head" or "just physical"; it's a recognition that such distinctions are artificially imposed on a human system that functions as an integrated whole.

When you recognize these connections, treatment becomes more effective and efficient. Breathing techniques that calm an anxious mind also reduce blood pressure. Processing traumatic experiences can resolve chronic pain that's resisted conventional treatment. Addressing nutritional deficiencies can alleviate depression symptoms. True healing happens when health problems aren't labeled as "just emotional" or "only physical" and are recognized as having distinct elements in both.

Breaking Down Mental Health Stigmas

Despite overwhelming evidence of mental health's centrality to overall well-being, stigma continues to prevent millions from seeking care. This stigma manifests itself in both subtle and overt ways from the language we use in everyday conversation to discriminatory practices that limit access to care.

The persistence of this stigma reflects deeply rooted misconceptions that have been remarkably resistant to change. First, the "moral weakness" myth is the false belief that mental health problems result from character flaws, lack of willpower, or moral failings rather than the complex interplay of biological, psychological, and environmental factors that actually drives these conditions. Another false assumption is that mental health challenges happen to "other people"—those who are different, weaker, or less capable—rather than that mental health is a universal human experience that affects people across all demographics. Finally, there is a misconception that mental health conditions are permanent character traits rather than treatable medical conditions that respond well to appropriate interventions.

These beliefs create barriers to care that wouldn't be tolerated for any other health condition. We don't tell people with diabetes to "just think positive thoughts" or suggest that heart disease patients should "pull themselves together," yet these harmful responses remain common for mental health struggles. The words we use matter profoundly in either perpetuating or dismantling mental health stigma. Common phrases such as "That's crazy," "She's being dramatic," "He's having a breakdown," and "Pull yourself together" minimize real suffering and reinforce harmful myths about mental health.

More damaging still is the tendency to use diagnostic terms casually: "I'm so OCD about organizing," "The weather is so bipolar," or "My boss is such a narcissist." This linguistic habit trivializes serious medical conditions and contributes to misunderstanding what these diagnoses actually involve. Professional settings often perpetuate stigma through euphemisms that distance us from a direct acknowledgment of mental health—"personal issues," "stress-related problems," or "work-life balance challenges"—rather than clearly naming depression, anxiety, or other specific conditions that deserve the same direct acknowledgment we give to diabetes or hypertension.

The tide is gradually turning, particularly among younger generations, who speak about therapy, anxiety, and depression with a candor that would have been unimaginable even two decades ago. Athletes openly discuss their mental health struggles. Celebrities share their experiences with therapy and medication. Workplaces increasingly acknowledge the importance of mental well-being.

This cultural shift represents more than increased awareness; it reflects a growing recognition of mental health as an essential component of human flourishing rather than an unfortunate affliction affecting "others." Social media, despite its many problems, has created platforms for authentic storytelling about mental health experiences that help normalize these universal human struggles. Yet room for progress remains.

Combating Stigma: What Works

Reducing mental health stigma requires more than awareness campaigns and celebrity endorsements. It demands structural changes that demonstrate genuine commitment to treating mental health as health:

- **Policy changes:** True insurance parity that ensures equal access to mental healthcare, workplace policies that accommodate mental health needs without penalty, and educational initiatives that teach emotional literacy from early childhood.
- **Integration into primary care:** When mental health services are woven seamlessly into general healthcare rather than segregated into separate "behavioral health" systems, it reinforces the understanding that mental health is simply health.
- **Personal responsibility:** Each of us has a role in examining our own biases and language choices. This means recognizing when we use stigmatizing language, challenging misconceptions when we encounter them, and modeling the understanding that seeking mental healthcare is a sign of wisdom and self-care, not weakness.

Perhaps most important, breaking down stigma requires all of us to move beyond abstract support for "mental health awareness" to concrete actions that demonstrate our belief that mental health is health. This might mean:

- Supporting colleagues who need mental health accommodations
- Choosing healthcare providers who demonstrate an integrated understanding of mind-body connections

- Advocating for mental health resources in our communities and workplaces
- Modeling appropriate language and attitudes in our daily interactions
- Teaching children that emotions and mental health are normal topics of conversation, not shameful secrets

When you truly internalize that mental health is health, you create space for the authentic conversations that lead to healing, connection, and integrated well-being.

The Most Common Mental Health Issue: Anxiety Disorders

We are wired for survival. Anxiety evolved as a protective mechanism, alerting us to potential dangers and preparing our bodies to respond. Your amygdala, the brain's threat detection center, doesn't distinguish between a saber-toothed tiger and a troubling CNN headline. Both trigger the same physiological cascade: elevated heart rate, shallow breathing, muscle tension, and a flood of stress hormones such as cortisol and adrenaline. This response is brilliantly designed to deal with immediate physical threats that require quick action. It's far less helpful when the "threat" is an endless scroll of global crises on your phone or a vague sense that something terrible might happen tomorrow.

What makes anxiety particularly challenging is that these responses aren't entirely irrational. The world does contain real dangers. But when anxiety becomes chronic, it stops serving its protective function and starts becoming the problem itself. As I often tell my patients with health-related anxiety: Sometimes the anxiety becomes the cancer. From a strictly medical perspective, anxiety disorders represent a dysregulation of normal stress responses. However, I've found this framing alone rarely helps my patients. The experience of anxiety isn't just biological—it's deeply psychological and contextual.

When I talk with patients about anxiety, I encourage them to consider three dimensions:

- **The physiological dimension:** What's happening in your body (racing heart, shallow breathing, muscle tension, sweaty palms, upset stomach)?
- **The cognitive dimension:** What's happening in your mind (worried thoughts, catastrophizing, rumination, marinating in "What ifs")?
- **The behavioral dimension:** How are you responding to these experiences (avoidance, reassurance seeking, distraction, self-medicating with substances, etc.)?

All three dimensions are important, because each offers different entry points for intervention. Some patients find relief by starting with the body, using breathing techniques or exercise to calm the physiological arousal. Others need to begin with their thoughts, identifying and challenging catastrophic thinking patterns. Still others benefit most from behavioral changes, such as limiting their media consumption or reconnecting with routines that provide structure amid chaos.

Michelle came to see me with what she described as "out-of-control anxiety." An executive in her mid-fifties, she typically managed stress well; she even prided herself on it. Her colleagues often remarked at her composure during high-stakes presentations and before impossible deadlines. But something had recently shifted. She found herself waking at 3:00 a.m. with her heart racing, checking news headlines compulsively throughout the day, and getting into tense arguments with her adult daughter over politics at family dinners. When her college-age son called to ask for advice about his roommate situation, she found herself catastrophizing about his entire future instead of offering the measured counsel she normally would.

"I've always been the steady one," she told me, her voice tight as she twisted the tissue in her hands. "But now I feel like I'm coming apart." She went on to describe her worries about everything happening in the world: wars, political division, climate disasters, plus concerns about retirement security and her mother's declining health. She reported having had to mute herself during a Zoom board meeting because she couldn't catch her breath. "I feel completely overwhelmed."

That sentence stuck with me, because I hear variations of it regularly. Many of my patients feel undone by anxiety. They wonder if persistent worry is just the admission price for living in today's world or if there is something medically wrong with them. Like Michelle, many people I see don't meet the full criteria for an anxiety disorder but are still significantly distressed. They exist in what we might call the "middle ground" of anxiety—not incapacitated but living with enough background anxiety that it interferes with their quality of life.

In clinical practice, we often work with categories and thresholds: Does this person meet the diagnostic criteria for generalized anxiety disorder? Is this level of distress clinically significant? These distinctions can be helpful for treatment decisions, but they don't always capture the lived experience of anxiety. Some clinicians will use the General Anxiety Disorder–7 (GAD-7) questionnaire to understand the patient's degree of distress, but for someone like Michelle, the GAD-7 questionnaire wouldn't flag her distress; it might actually cause a doctor (or a doctor's AI program) to dismiss it.

The reality is more nuanced. Anxiety exists on a spectrum, not as an either/or proposition. Each of us has a baseline level of vigilance, and we move along this continuum depending on our circumstances, resilience factors, and coping resources. Some amount of anxiety is adaptive, even productive. You need a little adrenaline to file your taxes on time! But too much becomes problematic. And the point at which it crosses from helpful to harmful varies tremendously from person to person.

During challenging times—a global pandemic, political upheaval, or a personal crisis—even those with typically robust mental health may find themselves experiencing more anxiety than usual. This doesn't necessarily mean that something is "wrong" with them; it might simply reflect a normal response to abnormal circumstances. Conversely, just because you can point to a cause for your anxiety doesn't mean that you don't need support.

Consider Lexi, who came to me concerned about her health after several specialists had dismissed her persistent gastrointestinal symptoms as "just anxiety." "Maybe it is all in my head," she said tearfully. "Everyone keeps telling me my tests are normal." Despite her having been labeled a hypochondriac, further investigation revealed that she had Crohn's disease, an inflammatory condition of the intestines. Her worry wasn't irrational; it was an appropriate response to real physical symptoms that hadn't been properly diagnosed. Once we addressed the underlying condition, her anxiety resolved because it had served its purpose: to alert her that something was genuinely wrong.

At the other end of the spectrum was Sarah, a young professional who cycled through seven specialists for complaints ranging from headaches and back pain to heart palpitations and hand tremors. Her medical chart was thick with normal test results and specialist referrals. What no one had recognized was that her physical symptoms weren't separate problems but manifestations of a significant anxiety disorder. Her racing thoughts triggered muscle tension, which caused headaches and back pain. Her fear of those symptoms created more anxiety, which manifested itself as palpitations. Rather than addressing that underlying pattern, the specialists had unknowingly reinforced it by ordering ever more tests and treatments for individual symptoms without addressing the integrated whole.

The distinction between helpful vigilance and problematic anxiety isn't always clear cut. Many people exist in a gray area in which anxiety isn't completely debilitating but still significantly impacts their quality of life. They may not meet formal diagnostic criteria but would nonetheless benefit from support. Recognizing where you fall on this spectrum isn't about labeling yourself but about understanding when and how to seek appropriate care.

When to Seek Professional Help

When should you worry about your mental health? What should you do about it? The answers to these questions are not always intuitive or easy.

You might ask yourself, "Am I mentally struggling? Or is this just a rough patch?" You might tell yourself things such as "Life is hard—of course I feel [depressed/anxious/out of control/alone]." You might convince yourself "Once I get past this [work project/family event/relationship problem], I will be fine."

Sometimes it is just a rough patch. Sometimes anxiety or sadness or rage appropriately matches the moment. Sometimes your problems are purely situational. But when the rough patch turns into a series of rough patches—or when the stressful situation finally passes and we're still not okay—it's time to ask yourself, "If this were a physical symptom—for example, a nagging cough or a bad headache—would I ask for help?" If the answer is yes, it may be time to seek professional attention.

Tolerance of distress varies from person to person. Some people can't pay attention to their needs until they're completely undone. Others become alarmed by a new bodily symptom or by sensing other people's discomfort. Others are blissfully unaware of how their anxiety or substance use affects other people.

While everyday fluctuations in mood and emotion are normal, certain patterns warrant professional attention. Consider seeking help if:

- Your emotional distress significantly impairs your daily functioning, making it difficult for you to work, maintain relationships, or care for yourself.
- Your symptoms persist longer than would be expected given the circumstances—such as grief that remains intensely debilitating years after a loss or anxiety that continues long after a stressful situation has resolved.

- You experience concerning changes in sleep, appetite, energy, or concentration that significantly deviate from your baseline.
- Your thoughts or behaviors become increasingly rigid or repetitive, such as compulsive checking (e.g., repeatedly verifying that home locks are secure, that stove burners are off, that car doors are locked), excessive hand washing, or severely restricted eating patterns.
- You develop thoughts about harming yourself or others, even if you have no intention of acting on them.
- You find yourself increasingly relying on substances to manage emotions or get through the day.
- Your friends or family express concern about changes in your behavior or emotional state that you may not fully recognize yourself.
- You feel stuck in patterns that you intellectually recognize as unhelpful but can't seem to change through willpower alone.

These guidelines aren't about pathologizing normal human struggles but about recognizing when professional support might help navigate particularly challenging mental health experiences. Many people benefit from therapy or medical intervention long before they reach a crisis point—often when they first notice patterns that affect their quality of life or relationships.

Take, for example, my patient Francesca, whose lab work was amiss at her annual checkup. She reported being off her usual exercise and eating routines. She hadn't refilled her thyroid and heart medications in months. However, the real problem wasn't her abnormal blood tests; she was struggling with debilitating anxiety. It turned out that taking a new position at her company had rekindled some deep insecurities about her competency and belonging. Anxious thoughts not only occupied a significant amount of her brain space, impairing her ability to sleep and maintain focus on the job; they were also negatively affecting her health.

The root cause of her physical complaints and abnormal lab tests was debilitating anxiety. The combination of worry and poor self-care had conspired to make her sick. When she realized that her anxiety was negatively affecting her health, she admitted that "powering through" was not an appropriate response to her situation.

Strategies to Treat Mental Health Problems

There is no one-size-fits-all prescription for better mental health. Whereas one person with alcohol dependence might need AA to get sober, another might need a divorce. Whereas one person's anxiety would improve with Zoloft, another would benefit from quitting coffee and engaging in meditation. Whereas one person's depression might lift with grief counseling, another's might abate with hormone replacement therapy.

When mental health challenges arise, taking meaningful action involves a balance of self-awareness, acceptance, and practical strategies. This approach isn't about "fixing" problems but about developing a more compassionate, effective relationship with your mind and emotions.

Recognize Your Patterns

The first step is developing awareness of your unique mental health patterns. This means noticing:

- **Your personal triggers:** What consistently leads to deteriorating mental health for you? Certain relationships, environments, physical states, or thought patterns? Identifying these patterns helps you anticipate and prepare for challenging situations.
- **Your physical manifestations:** How does mental distress show up in your body? Common physical indicators include sleep changes, appetite shifts, muscle tension, digestive issues, and energy fluctuations. These bodily signals often appear before conscious recognition of emotional changes.

- **Your thought patterns:** What narratives dominate your thinking when you are struggling? Do you catastrophize, overgeneralize, personalize, or engage in black-and-white thinking? These cognitive patterns shape your emotional experience and behavioral choices.
- **Your behavioral responses:** What do you do when feeling emotionally challenged? Do you withdraw, seek connection, scroll social media sites endlessly, overwork, undersleep, or change your eating patterns? Recognizing these behaviors will help you interrupt unhelpful coping mechanisms before they deepen your distress.

This self-awareness isn't about self-judgment; it's about creating a map of your mental health landscape so you can navigate it more effectively. The goal isn't to eliminate uncomfortable feelings but to develop a more conscious relationship with them.

Meet Yourself Where You Are

Once you've developed an awareness of your patterns, the next step involves acceptance—not resignation but a clear-eyed, nonjudgmental recognition of your current reality.

- **Accept that mental health fluctuations are part of being human.** Our emotional systems developed to respond to changing circumstances, both external and internal. Expecting constant stability creates suffering when natural variations occur.
- **Accept where you are right now.** Fighting against your current reality—telling yourself "I shouldn't feel this way" or "I need to get over this immediately"—creates a secondary layer of suffering. Accepting your present experience doesn't mean approving of it or believing that it will last forever.

- **Accept what you can and cannot control.** Much mental distress stems from attempting to control what's beyond our influence: other people's behavior, past events, or an uncertain future. Clarity about your sphere of influence helps you redirect energy toward taking actionable steps rather than ruminating.

I remember a patient named Jamie who came to me for heart palpitations. After ruling out cardiac issues, we identified anxiety as the driver. She described lying awake nightly, imagining worst-case scenarios for her children, her health, and world events. What helped wasn't dismissing those concerns but acknowledging that they reflected her deep care for her family and her world while recognizing her limited ability to control those domains.

Take Meaningful Action

The final step involves developing agency—taking meaningful action within your sphere of influence. This isn't about eliminating difficult emotions entirely but about building a more constructive relationship with them.

Physiological interventions that can help regulate your nervous system include:

- Deep breathing techniques emphasizing longer exhalations, which activate the parasympathetic "rest and digest" response
- Regular physical movement, which releases tension and stress hormones
- Adequate sleep, nutrition, and hydration, which provide the physiological foundation for emotional regulation
- Limiting your intake of stimulants such as caffeine and depressants such as alcohol that can increase your emotional volatility

Cognitive strategies that can help manage your thought patterns include:

- Challenging catastrophic thinking by asking "What's the evidence?" and "What's most likely to happen?"
- Practicing thought diffusion—observing thoughts without identifying with them
- Setting boundaries around media consumption and information intake
- Developing realistic contingency plans for legitimate concerns rather than endlessly worrying

Behavioral approaches that can create structural support include:

- Establishing routines that provide predictability during uncertain times
- Building in pleasurable activities and meaningful connection that buffer against stress
- Setting boundaries with people or situations that consistently trigger distress
- Getting an accountability partner or working with professional allies for more severe challenges

For Jamie, gaining agency involved setting a media curfew (no news after 7:00 p.m.), establishing a wind-down routine with calming activities, learning diaphragmatic breathing techniques, and scheduling regular times to discuss her concerns with her partner rather than ruminating alone at night. Those changes didn't eliminate her anxiety completely, but they created enough space around it that it no longer dominated her life.

Ask for Professional Help

Psychotherapy provides structured support for processing difficult emotions, changing unhelpful thought patterns, and developing new coping skills. Evidence-based approaches such as cognitive behavioral therapy (CBT), acceptance and commitment therapy (ACT), and psychodynamic therapy have strong research support for various mental health conditions. The therapeutic relationship itself—feeling truly heard and understood by someone who isn't personally involved in your situation—often provides significant healing.

Medication can be an important tool for addressing biological aspects of mental health conditions. For some people, particularly those with severe depression, bipolar disorder, or treatment-resistant anxiety, medication provides the stabilization necessary for other therapeutic approaches to work effectively. Modern psychiatric medications, while not perfect, have improved substantially in recent decades, with more targeted approaches and better side effect profiles than earlier generations of drugs.

Integrative approaches combining multiple treatment modalities often prove most effective, especially for complex or long-standing issues. These might include therapy and medication management alongside lifestyle modifications, support groups, mind-body practices such as yoga or meditation, and sometimes alternative approaches such as acupuncture or nutritional intervention.

The mental health strategies discussed—exercise, social connection, stress management—also provide powerful support for cognitive function. We'll examine these connections more deeply in chapter 13, where we will focus specifically on caring for your brain's thinking, memory, and attention systems.

Finding the Right Mental Health Help

The process of finding appropriate mental health support can feel overwhelming, especially when you're already struggling. Some practical steps include:

- Start with your primary care provider, who can provide an initial assessment, potential medication options, and referrals to mental health specialists.

- Check with your insurance provider for covered mental health professionals in your area or telehealth options.
- Explore resources such as *Psychology Today*'s therapist directory, which allows filtering by location, specialty, insurance, and treatment approach.
- Consider online therapy platforms that offer more accessible options, particularly for those in rural areas or with mobility challenges.
- For immediate support during crisis situations, resources such as the 988 Suicide & Crisis Lifeline provide 24/7 assistance.

Remember: Finding the right therapeutic match often requires some trial and error. It's entirely appropriate to have consultation appointments with several providers before committing to ongoing work or to change provider if the relationship doesn't feel helpful after several sessions.

Mental Health's Role in Physical Well-being

One of the most powerful yet overlooked aspects of mental health is its role in physical healing. When you are chronically stressed, anxious, or depressed, your body's heightened state of physiological arousal compromises every organ system, from digestive function to hormonal regulation. Addressing mental health issues isn't a luxury; it is necessary for overall health.

The Stress-Inflammation Connection

Chronic psychological stress directly increases inflammatory markers throughout the body. This inflammation, when persistent, contributes to nearly every major chronic disease from cardiovascular issues and diabetes to autoimmune conditions and even cancer progression.

Consider Leila, who came to me with persistent digestive issues that several gastroenterologists had attributed to IBS. Her symptoms flared dramatically during workweeks but improved during vacations, a pattern she herself had noticed but that previous doctors had dismissed. Further conversation revealed that she worked under a verbally abusive manager in a chronically understaffed department, creating constant fight-or-flight system activation. Her digestive system was literally shutting down in response to that ongoing threat.

While medication provided symptomatic relief, true healing required addressing the psychological safety issue at its root. With support from therapy and workplace advocacy resources, Leila eventually secured a transfer to another department. Her digestive symptoms improved dramatically—not because we found the right medication combination but because we removed the chronic threat response that was dysregulating her gut function.

The Protective Power of Mental Well-being

Your body's healing mechanisms function optimally in states of relative calm and safety. When you perceive a threat—whether from external circumstances or internal emotional distress—healing processes take a back seat to survival responses. This explains why chronic stress slows recovery from illness. Research has consistently demonstrated this connection: A comprehensive meta-analysis found that psychological stress is associated with significantly impaired wound healing.[5]

For patients recovering from surgery, injury, or acute illness, addressing mental health is fundamental for physical recovery. Simple interventions that increase psychological safety—clear communication about treatment plans, pain management that prevents suffering, and emotional support during recovery—significantly improve medical outcomes across virtually all conditions. I worked with Raj, a fifty-eight-year-old recovering from bypass surgery whose rehabilitation was progressing more slowly than expected. While his surgical team focused exclusively on physical

---

5 Jessica Walburn et al., "Psychological Stress and Wound Healing in Humans: A Systematic Review and Meta-Analysis," *Journal of Psychosomatic Research* 67 no. 3 (September 2009): 235–271, https://pubmed.ncbi.nlm.nih.gov/19686881/.

parameters, my conversations revealed his intense anxiety about job security. That anxiety was keeping his nervous system in a state of high alert, preventing the parasympathetic dominance needed for optimal healing. Once he got connected with HR and a financial planner and after learning basic relaxation techniques, his body began to heal.

Sturdy mental health serves as a protective buffer against the inevitable stressors and challenges of life. This resilience isn't about avoiding difficulties but about developing the internal resources to navigate them without becoming overwhelmed. People with robust mental health still experience pain, grief, anxiety, and other difficult emotions, but they recover more quickly and maintain perspective during challenging times.

Research consistently shows that psychological resilience factors—social connection, emotional regulation skills, a sense of purpose, and psychological flexibility—correlate with better health outcomes and longevity, even when controlling for traditional risk factors. A large-scale study tracking over 10,000 older adults found that for each standard deviation increase in psychological resilience, the risk of death decreased by 25 percent, even after adjusting for chronic diseases and health behaviors.[6] These mental resources literally change how your body responds to everything from viral infections to chronic disease.

Juanita, a seventy-two-year-old with multiple chronic conditions including arthritis and heart disease, surprised her specialists with her consistently stable health despite her advanced age and medical complexity. What they missed in their assessments was her extraordinary psychological resilience: her deep social connections, her daily gratitude practices, volunteer work that gave her purpose, and a remarkable ability to accept her limitations without being defined by them.

6 Xiang Wang et al., "Association of Psychological Resilience with All-Cause and Cause-Specific Mortality in Older Adults: A Cohort Study," *BMC Public Health* 24, 1989 (July 25, 2024), https://pubmed.ncbi.nlm.nih.gov/39054517/.

These psychological strengths didn't eliminate her medical conditions, but they created an internal environment in which her body could manage them more effectively. Her example illustrates how mental well-being doesn't just make you feel better; it fundamentally alters your physiological functioning in ways that promote health and enhance our quality of life. In the next chapter we will explore another important aspect of brain health: cognition.

13

Caring for Your Brain

Building on our exploration of mental health as the foundation of overall well-being, this chapter focuses specifically on cognitive health, the brain functions that enable you to think clearly, focus your attention, and make and retrieve memories. While intimately connected to the emotional well-being discussed in chapter 12, cognitive health is a distinct dimension of brain function with its own evidence-based care strategies and unique vulnerabilities.

Cognitive health encompasses far more than avoiding dementia or age-related decline, though these concerns motivate many people to pay attention to their brain health for the first time. Your cognitive abilities—attention and concentration, memory systems, processing speed, language skills, and executive functions such as planning and decision-making—influence every aspect of how you navigate daily life from managing your health information (your INFORMATICS quadrant) to making choices about what you consume (your INPUTS quadrant) to maintaining the physical practices that support your body (your INFRASTRUCTURE quadrant).

The mental health foundation established in chapter 12 directly influences cognitive function in profound ways. Anxiety can impair working memory and scatter attention across multiple worry streams. Depression affects processing speed and decision-making, creating the mental fog that many patients describe as feeling as though they're "thinking through molasses." Chronic stress keeps cognitive resources allocated to threat detection rather than available for the complex thinking, learning, and memory consolidation that define mental sharpness.

Understanding cognitive health as part of your complete health ecosystem helps explain why brain function varies so dramatically from person to person and even within the same person across different life phases. The executive stressed about work deadlines who can't concentrate on reading; the student whose attention fractures across social media, study materials, and text messages; the parent juggling many demands who feels that their memory isn't what it used to be; these experiences reflect not cognitive deficits but natural responses to environments and circumstances that challenge our brain's optimal operation.

When Cognitive Health Becomes a Hidden Driver

To understand how cognitive health affects your complete well-being, consider Walter's story. Walter had been one of my healthiest patients for years. At age seventy-nine, the retired high school history teacher was physically active, socially engaged with his weekly chess club, and sharp as a tack when discussing current events. He would arrive at appointments with a neatly organized folder containing his medication list, questions written on index cards, and a small notebook in which he tracked his blood pressure readings.

During his regular checkup last spring, however, I noticed subtle changes. His usually crisp, clean button-down shirt had a stain on the sleeve. His wife, Margaret, who typically waited in the lobby, had come into the exam room for the first time. When I asked about his blood pressure logs, he rummaged through his coat pockets before Margaret quietly leaned toward me. "I didn't want to worry you," she whispered while Walter was changing into a gown, "but Walter's been forgetting his medications. I've been trying to help, but I work part-time at the library, and I can't always be there to remind him."

Walter's vital signs that day were concerning: His blood pressure was 168/94 mmHg, significantly higher than his usual well-controlled readings of around 130/80 mmHg. His weight had dropped seven pounds since his last visit three months earlier. His lab work revealed vitamin deficiencies and worsening prediabetes. When I inquired about his diet, he confidently stated that he was "eating just fine," but Margaret's eyes told a different story. It was becoming clear that Walter's health issues weren't separate problems but symptoms of an underlying cognitive decline that was affecting his ability to manage his daily health routines.

I administered the Montreal Cognitive Assessment (MoCA), a ten-minute test, which confirmed my suspicions. Walter scored 21 out of 30, indicating mild cognitive impairment. He struggled particularly with the delayed recall section, executive function tasks, and orientation to time.

Walter's case illustrates a critical pattern I've observed repeatedly in my practice: Cognitive decline often manifests itself first as seemingly unrelated physical health problems. By recognizing cognitive impairment as the underlying driver rather than treating each symptom in isolation, we were able to implement a comprehensive care plan that addressed both the cause and its cascading effects. Six months later, Walter's physical health markers had improved with a comprehensive approach including medication management, nutritional support, and social services. While his cognitive assessment scores hadn't improved significantly, they hadn't worsened either, which was a victory in itself.

The Cognitive Engine: What's Under the Hood

Walter's experience demonstrates how cognitive health involves multiple interconnected systems that work together to support how you think and function. When these systems begin to falter, the effects ripple throughout your entire health ecosystem. Cognitive health encompasses much more than memory. What else is included in the whole brain package?

- **Attention and focus** are your brain's ability to concentrate on relevant information while filtering out distractions. This capacity includes sustaining attention over time—such as Walter's ability to track his blood pressure readings consistently—selecting what deserves focus amid competing demands and appropriately managing multiple tasks when necessary. This attention system is the foundation of all other cognitive functions, since you can't effectively remember, learn about, or solve problems without first directing cognitive resources toward the relevant information.

- **Memory systems** work in sophisticated coordination to help you navigate both immediate demands and long-term goals. Working memory holds information temporarily while you use it, such as remembering which medications to take when. This system has limited capacity and can become overwhelmed when you try to juggle too many pieces of information simultaneously. Short-term memory retains information for brief periods, while long-term memory stores and retrieves the vast repository of knowledge, experiences, and skills you've accumulated throughout your life.

- **Executive function** encompasses the higher-order cognitive skills that enable you to manage life's complexity. These are the abilities Walter was gradually losing that affected his medication adherence and self-care routines. They include planning and organization abilities, which help you sequence tasks and manage time effectively; decision-making and problem-solving skills, which enable you to weigh options and find solutions; cognitive flexibility, which allows you to adapt when circumstances change; and impulse control, which helps you align your actions with your long-term goals rather than your immediate desires.

- **Processing speed** affects how quickly your brain can take in, understand, and respond to information, influencing everything from conversation flow to complex task completion. Language skills include not just vocabulary and grammar but verbal fluency, comprehension, and the ability to find and use words effectively in communication. These cognitive dimensions don't operate in isolation but function as an integrated system, with each component supporting and being supported by the others.

Key Signs That Your Cognitive Health Needs Attention

- Difficulty completing tasks that used to feel automatic, such as managing medications or finances
- Increasing difficulty with multitasking or organizing complex activities
- Memory lapses that interfere with daily functioning rather than occasional forgetfulness
- Changes in language abilities, such as difficulty finding words or following conversations
- Personality changes, increased irritability, or shifts in judgment and decision-making
- Physical health problems that seem unrelated but coincide with cognitive changes

Remember: Cognitive changes can be the first sign of treatable conditions such as depression, sleep disorders, medication effects, or nutritional deficiencies. Don't dismiss symptoms as "just aging"; many cognitive issues can be improved with proper evaluation and intervention.

Beyond Memory Loss: Common Cognitive Challenges

When most people think about cognitive problems, memory loss comes to mind first, often accompanied by fears about dementia. While memory concerns deserve significant attention, many cognitive challenges stem from treatable conditions rather than progressive neurological diseases. Let's start with the big one first.

Dementia and Cognitive Impairment

Dementia is not a single disease but a syndrome characterized by progressive cognitive decline severe enough to interfere with daily functioning. Alzheimer's disease accounts for 60 to 80 percent of cases, but vascular dementia, Lewy body dementia, and frontotemporal dementia also contribute significantly to the approximately 10 percent of adults over sixty-five and nearly half of those over eighty-five who experience some form of cognitive impairment.

What many people don't realize is how dementia and cognitive impairment act as hidden drivers of other health problems, as Walter's case demonstrated. When cognitive function declines, the ability to manage medications, follow treatment plans, recognize symptoms, and make health decisions becomes compromised. This creates a cascade of consequences that can affect every aspect of physical and mental well-being—uncontrolled blood pressure from forgotten medications, weight loss from poor nutrition, social isolation from dropped activities, and worsening health metrics that seem unrelated to brain function.

The treatment approach for cognitive impairment must address this cascade comprehensively rather than treating each symptom in isolation. Sometimes the most significant improvements come not from cognitive interventions but from addressing the secondary health problems that cognitive decline creates, while simultaneously providing support systems that compensate for declining cognitive abilities.

Stroke and Vascular Events

Stroke is one of the most significant yet most frequently misunderstood causes of cognitive changes. While physical effects such as weakness and speech difficulties receive attention, the cognitive consequences often go unrecognized, particularly when they occur without dramatic physical symptoms.

Consider my patient Tabitha, a sixty-eight-year-old retired teacher concerned about her increasing difficulty finding words during conversation.

Her family noticed those lapses and worried that she might have dementia. What distinguished Tabitha's case was the pattern; her word-finding difficulties had appeared suddenly after what she described as "a terrible migraine" six months earlier, rather than gradually worsening over time.

When I explored that history, Tabitha recalled that during the "migraine," she had experienced about thirty minutes when her speech had been slurred and she had felt confused—symptoms she had dismissed once her headache had subsided. Neuroimaging revealed damage in her left temporal lobe consistent with a past stroke, likely occurring during the episode she had attributed to a migraine. With that diagnosis, we offered Tabitha targeted speech therapy specifically designed for poststroke aphasia rather than treatments for progressive dementia. We also implemented stroke prevention measures to reduce her risk of future events. Unlike the gradual decline seen in conditions such as Alzheimer's, stroke typically produces sudden, noticeable cognitive changes. Depending on its location in the brain, a stroke might affect language processing, visual-spatial awareness, memory, or executive function while leaving other cognitive domains intact.

Stroke-related cognitive changes often occur in people with vascular risk factors—hypertension, diabetes, high cholesterol, smoking—that may have been present for years, creating vulnerability long before symptoms emerge. Even "silent" strokes can damage neural pathways critical to thinking and memory, accumulating over time to cause significant cognitive impairment without obvious physical symptoms.

Perhaps most important, stroke is one of the most preventable causes of cognitive impairment. Managing vascular risk factors significantly reduces stroke risk, while prompt medical evaluation for even transient neurological symptoms can preserve cognitive function that might otherwise be permanently lost.

Often Overlooked Factors Affecting Cognition

Several other factors significantly impact cognitive function yet frequently go unrecognized in healthcare settings, leading to missed opportunities for intervention and improvement.

Hearing Loss

Nearly two-thirds of adults over age seventy have some degree of hearing loss, yet it often goes undiagnosed and untreated. This sensory deficit affects far more than just their communication; it has direct implications for their brain health. Research has established a clear link between untreated hearing loss and accelerated cognitive decline.

When you struggle to hear conversations, your brain diverts cognitive resources from memory and thinking to the effortful task of deciphering sounds. Over time, this cognitive overload can contribute to neural changes. Additionally, hearing difficulties often lead to social withdrawal, which removes valuable cognitive stimulation and can contribute to depression—both risk factors for cognitive decline.

The encouraging news is that addressing hearing loss can help. Studies suggest that hearing aid use is associated with better cognitive performance and may slow cognitive decline. Yet despite this evidence, only about 20 percent of people who could benefit from hearing aids actually use them, often due to stigma, cost, or limited access to hearing healthcare.

Grief and Emotional Distress

The stress responses we explored in chapter 12—the fight-flight-freeze reactions that protect us from danger—can become problematic when chronically activated. Persistent stress hormones that maintain emotional vigilance also impair the cognitive functions we rely on for complex thinking, learning, and memory formation. Grief, depression, anxiety, and chronic stress can all impair cognitive performance in ways that mimic dementia.

Consider my patient Lila, who came to me six months after her daughter's sudden death. Her husband was concerned about possible dementia; Lila was forgetting appointments, misplacing items, and struggling to follow conversations. A cognitive assessment revealed difficulties with attention and working memory, but not the pattern typical of Alzheimer's disease. What she was experiencing was "pseudodementia"—cognitive impairment secondary to depression and grief. Her emotional pain was so consuming that it left her little cognitive capacity for everyday tasks. With appropriate treatment for depression and grief support, her cognitive symptoms gradually improved over several months. This connection works in the other direction as well; cognitive changes can trigger or worsen emotional distress, creating a vicious cycle that requires addressing the cognitive and emotional dimensions simultaneously.

Sleep Disorders

Sleep is perhaps the most undervalued pillar of brain health. During sleep, especially deep sleep, your brain clears out metabolic waste products, consolidates memories, and repairs neural connections. Disrupted sleep patterns, even in the short term, can significantly impair cognitive function.

Chronic sleep problems are particularly concerning for cognitive health. Sleep apnea, which affects up to 30 percent of older adults, causes repeated oxygen deprivation during sleep and is strongly linked to cognitive impairment. Other sleep disorders, including insomnia and REM sleep behavior disorder, also correlate with an increased risk of cognitive decline.

Even without a diagnosable sleep disorder, insufficient or poor-quality sleep takes a toll on cognition. Many people accept chronic sleep deprivation as normal in our busy world, not recognizing how it compromises their thinking, memory, and decision-making capacities.

Medication Effects

Many commonly prescribed medications can affect cognitive function, often in ways that patients and even providers fail to recognize. Anticholinergic medications (found in many over-the-counter sleep aids, allergy medications, and bladder control drugs) are particularly problematic, as they block a neurotransmitter important for memory and thinking.

Other medications with potential cognitive side effects include certain antidepressants, anxiolytics, anticonvulsants, and pain medications. In older adults, even appropriate doses can accumulate to problematic levels due to age-related changes in metabolism and elimination. The risk increases substantially when a person is taking more than one medication simultaneously, which is common among older adults. Each additional medication increases the potential for interactions that might affect brain function.

Head Injuries and Traumatic Brain Injury

Head injuries are one of the most underappreciated factors affecting cognitive function. From seemingly minor concussions to severe traumatic brain injuries (TBIs), head trauma can create lasting cognitive changes that often go undiagnosed or are minimized, particularly when they occur outside sports or military contexts.

Even a single concussion can disrupt the neural networks supporting attention, memory, and executive function. The brain's delicate tissue can suffer microscopic damage that may not appear on standard imaging yet can significantly alter cognitive processing. What makes concussions particularly concerning is their cumulative effect. Research shows that multiple concussions, even mild ones separated by years, can compound their impact on cognitive function, each injury potentially lowering the threshold for subsequent damage while reducing the brain's recovery capacity.

Consider my patient Derek, a forty-two-year-old construction manager who came to me complaining of "brain fog," irritability, and difficulty concentrating. Initial screenings for depression, sleep disorders, and thyroid dysfunction revealed nothing significant. It wasn't until I asked about past head injuries that a pattern emerged. Derek had experienced what he described as "just a few bumps on the head" throughout his life—a bicycle accident at twelve, a car collision in his twenties, and two incidents at construction sites. None had resulted in hospitalization, and he'd prided himself on "walking them off." Yet those seemingly disconnected events had created a cumulative burden of neurological injury that was now manifesting itself as cognitive symptoms.

Neuropsychological testing confirmed deficits in Derek's working memory, attention switching, and emotional regulation—all consistent with repeated mild traumatic brain injuries. Having that information transformed Derek's understanding of his symptoms from mysterious cognitive decline to a recognizable pattern with specific management strategies.

What makes head injuries particularly challenging is their often invisible nature. Unlike a broken bone that shows on an X-ray, concussion effects frequently manifest themselves through subtle changes in thinking, emotional regulation, and sensory processing. Patients may struggle to articulate these changes, particularly when they evolve slowly over time. The long-term consequences can be substantial. Research on chronic traumatic encephalopathy (CTE) has highlighted the potential connection between repeated head trauma and neurodegenerative disease. While most concussion patients won't develop CTE, many experience persistent cognitive challenges affecting their quality of life.

We need to change the cultural narrative around "toughing it out" after head injuries. The outdated notion that one should simply "shake off" a concussion can create lasting neurological harm. Instead, we should encourage reporting symptoms and following proper recovery protocols without stigma. For patients with unexplained cognitive symptoms, exploring the possibility of past head injuries—even those that seemed minor at the time—may reveal crucial insights for diagnosis and treatment that standard medical procedures often miss.

Where to Get Help for Cognitive Issues

While lifestyle factors significantly influence cognitive health, professional support plays an essential role, particularly when concerns arise. Knowing when and how to access care can make the difference between early intervention and missed opportunities.

Primary care providers can conduct initial screenings such as the Mini–Mental State Examination (MMSE) or Montreal Cognitive Assessment (MoCA) to evaluate cognitive function. These tools assess orientation, memory, attention, language, and visuospatial skills. While not diagnostic on their own, they provide valuable information about whether further evaluation is warranted.

For more comprehensive assessment, neuropsychological testing conducted by a specialized psychologist provides detailed information about specific cognitive domains. This testing can distinguish among different causes of cognitive symptoms and identify strengths as well as areas of concern.

Beyond assessment, various specialists may be involved in cognitive care.

- **Neurologists** focus on brain and nervous system disorders.
- **Geriatricians** specialize in the comprehensive care of older adults.
- **Psychiatrists** address cognitive symptoms related to mental health conditions.
- **Occupational therapists** help develop strategies to maintain function and independence.
- **Speech-language pathologists** assist with communication and cognitive rehabilitation.
- **Social workers** connect patients and families with resources and support services.

Navigating this complex landscape often requires advocacy—for yourself or for loved ones. Don't hesitate to seek second opinions, ask for recommendations, and ensure that your values and preferences remain central to your care decisions.

Modern Challenges to Cognitive Health

Beyond medical causes of cognitive changes, our brains face unprecedented challenges from the information-rich, distraction-heavy environment of modern life. Many patients come to me with attention difficulties, memory concerns, and "brain fog" that don't stem from underlying neurological conditions but rather from the unprecedented demands our modern environment places on our cognitive systems. Understanding these challenges helps distinguish between symptoms that need medical attention and those that can be addressed through lifestyle modifications and environmental changes.

The most pervasive challenge involves what researchers call "continuous partial attention": constantly monitoring multiple information streams without fully engaging with any single task. We check email while listening to podcasts, scroll social media during television shows, and attempt to do complex work while monitoring notifications. This has become so normalized that many people no longer recognize focused attention as a distinct cognitive state.

Research demonstrates that the mere presence of a smartphone (even when turned off!) can reduce cognitive performance on tasks requiring sustained attention. This "brain drain" effect occurs because part of our cognitive resources remains allocated to resisting the urge to check the device. The constant availability of stimulating content trains our brains to expect novelty frequently, making sustained focus feel increasingly uncomfortable.

This challenge particularly affects young people, whose brains develop during a period of intense digital exposure. The adolescent brain, still forming attention and impulse control networks, becomes accustomed to rapid task switching and frequent dopamine hits from social media interactions. Studies show that adolescents who spend more than three hours daily on social media have significantly higher rates of attention problems, with consequences for their academic performance and social development.

What makes digital distraction particularly concerning is the way it mimics other cognitive conditions. A teenager struggling with attention due to excessive screen time might be misdiagnosed with ADHD. An adult experiencing mental fatigue from constant multitasking might worry about early dementia. These misattributions create unnecessary anxiety and can lead to inappropriate treatments.

The attention challenges created by constant connectivity often connect to unconscious patterns that we'll explore in chapter 14. Compulsive phone checking, difficulty sustaining focus, and anxiety when separated from devices frequently stem from deeper beliefs about productivity, connection, and self-worth that operate beneath conscious awareness.

Practical Strategies to Reclaim Your Attention in a Distracted World

The good news is that your attention capacity is remarkably responsive to environmental changes. Here are some evidence-based approaches for protecting and strengthening this vital cognitive resource.

- **Create attention sanctuaries.** Designate specific times and spaces where digital interruptions are eliminated. This might mean a phone-free bedroom, screen-free meals, or a workspace in which notifications are disabled. These sanctuaries allow your attention system to recover from the constant vigilance required by our connected environment.
- **Practice single-tasking.** Despite the cultural glorification of multitasking, cognitive science clearly demonstrates that the human brain doesn't truly multitask; it switches rapidly between tasks, with each switch carrying a cognitive cost. Intentionally focusing on one activity at a time—whether work, conversation, or even leisure—strengthens your attention networks and increases both efficiency and enjoyment.
- **Implement digital boundaries.** Specific techniques such as time blocking (designating specific periods to check email and social media), app limits (using built-in phone features to restrict usage), and notification management (limiting alerts to truly time-sensitive matters) can dramatically reduce attention fragmentation.

- **Engage in attention training.** Activities that require sustained focus—reading physical books, practicing mindfulness meditation, engaging in flow-inducing hobbies such as crafting or playing music—act as "cognitive weightlifting" for attention muscles. Even brief daily periods of deep focus can strengthen the neural networks that support sustained attention.
- **Monitor your digital nutrition.** Just as we consider the nutritional value of food, we can evaluate our information consumption. Ask: Does this content enrich my understanding, inspire creativity, or meaningfully connect me with others? Or does it primarily trigger outrage, anxiety, or passive consumption? Curating higher-quality information inputs often leads to improved cognitive outcomes.
- **Understand the vulnerability window.** Research suggests that the first and last hours of the day are particularly important for cognitive function. Many people reach for their phones immediately upon waking and right before sleeping, exposing their brains to stimulating content and blue light at precisely the times when the brain most needs a calm transition. Creating phone-free morning and evening routines can significantly improve both attention and sleep quality.

For adolescents, these strategies are even more critical as their developing brains are particularly sensitive to attention disruption. Parents can model healthy technology use, create family-wide digital boundaries, and ensure that teens have access to engaging offline activities that promote sustained attention and social connection.

By understanding attention as a finite, precious resource—one that requires protection and cultivation in our distraction-rich world—you can maintain this vital cognitive function throughout life, supporting not just performance but a deeper engagement with what matters to you most.

The Six Pillars of Brain Health

Cognitive health isn't determined by genetics alone, though genetic factors certainly influence baseline cognitive abilities and vulnerability to cognitive decline. The everyday choices you make significantly influence how well your brain functions now and how well it will age over time. Understanding the evidence-based approaches to protecting and enhancing cognitive function provides a foundation for making informed decisions about brain health throughout your lifespan.

The following six pillars are based on the most robust scientific evidence for supporting cognitive health. Notice how each pillar connects not only to brain function but to your complete health ecosystem, illustrating the integrated nature of optimal well-being.

Pillar 1: Exercise: Moving for Your Mind

As discussed in the INFRASTRUCTURE quadrant, movement is medicine. Among all lifestyle factors, physical activity consistently emerges as one of the most powerful protectors of cognitive health. Regular exercise benefits the brain by improving blood flow and oxygen delivery to the brain; stimulating the production of growth factors that support neuronal health and neurogenesis; reducing inflammation and oxidative stress; enhancing the brain's ability to form new connections (neuroplasticity); improving sleep quality; and reducing risk factors for dementia, including hypertension, diabetes, and obesity.

The most robust evidence supports aerobic exercises that increase heart rate and breathing, such as walking, swimming, cycling, and dancing. However, resistance training also shows benefits for cognitive function, particularly for executive functions such as planning and multitasking.

The good news is that you don't need to become a marathon runner to see cognitive benefits. Studies suggest that even moderate activity, like brisk walking for thirty minutes several times a week, can improve cognitive performance and reduce dementia risk. The key is consistency and enjoyment. The best exercise regimen is one you'll maintain over time, so finding activities you enjoy is crucial for long-term brain health.

Pillar 2: Nutrition: Feeding Your Mind

The nutrition strategies discussed in the INPUTS quadrant directly affect your brain health. The antioxidants that protect cognitive function, the processed foods that impair attention, the caffeine that enhances alertness but disrupts sleep—all demonstrate how your cognitive health depends on conscious input choices. Your brain is a metabolically demanding organ, consuming about 20 percent of your body's calories despite making up only 2 percent of your body weight, which is why it makes sense that the quality of fuel you provide it directly impacts how well it functions.

Research increasingly supports the Mediterranean and Mediterranean-DASH Intervention for Neurodegenerative Delay (MIND) diets for brain health. These eating patterns emphasize vegetables (especially leafy greens), fruits (particularly berries), whole grains, fish and seafood, olive oil, and nuts and seeds while limiting the consumption of red meat and alcohol.

These diets are rich in anti-inflammatory compounds and nutrients that support brain function. They're also associated with reduced risk factors for cognitive decline, including cardiovascular disease, diabetes, and obesity. While no single food or supplement provides a magic bullet for brain health, the overall pattern of eating nutritious, minimally processed foods that support cardiovascular health also supports cognitive function.

Pillar 3: Good-Quality Sleep: Your Brain's Maintenance System

Sleep is the brain's primary maintenance and restoration period, when crucial processes occur that cannot happen during waking hours. During sleep, your brain consolidates memories, transferring important information from temporary storage into your long-term memory system while clearing away unnecessary information that would otherwise create cognitive clutter. The brain's glymphatic system becomes particularly active during sleep, clearing away metabolic waste products including the amyloid plaques associated with Alzheimer's disease.

Sleep also restores neurotransmitter balance, processes emotional experiences, and provides the neural recovery necessary for optimal cognitive performance the following day. Chronic sleep deprivation impairs virtually every aspect of cognitive function; attention becomes scattered, working memory capacity decreases, decision-making suffers, and emotional regulation becomes more difficult. These effects help explain why sleep problems often appear in your health data through changes in mood, stress hormone levels, and inflammatory markers. Sleep isn't a luxury; it's cognitive maintenance.

Pillar 4: Social Connection: Interpersonal Engagement as Brain Food

Social engagement also plays a crucial role in cognitive health. Longitudinal studies consistently show that people with stronger social ties have better cognitive outcomes as they age, including lower rates of dementia and slower cognitive decline.

Social connection provides cognitive stimulation that no individual mental exercise can replicate. Human brains evolved for social interaction, and maintaining meaningful relationships challenges several cognitive systems simultaneously while providing the emotional support that reduces stress and promotes overall brain health. Engaging in conversations requires real-time language processing, working memory, attention control, and theory of mind—the ability to understand others' perspectives and mental states.

Quality matters more than quantity when it comes to social connection and cognitive health. Deep, supportive relationships that involve regular meaningful interaction provide more cognitive benefit than do numerous superficial social contacts. Conversely, negative, stressful, or coercive relationships may increase cognitive risk through chronic stress activation. This helps explain why loneliness has been identified as a significant risk factor for cognitive decline, while strong social networks appear to be protective against dementia and other age-related cognitive changes.

The goal isn't to maintain constant connection with everyone but to engage meaningfully in relationships that support your authentic self while respecting others' boundaries and needs.

Pillar 5: Mental Stimulation: Use It or Lose It

Mental stimulation through engaging in cognitively challenging activities promotes neuroplasticity, the brain's remarkable ability to form new connections and adapt throughout life. However, not all mental activities provide equal cognitive benefit. Effective mental stimulation involves learning new skills rather than repeating familiar ones, challenges several cognitive domains simultaneously, adapts to your improving abilities over time, and engages both analytical and creative thinking processes.

Learning a new language exemplifies this type of beneficial cognitive challenge; it requires attention control, memory, pattern recognition, and executive function while providing the satisfaction of meaningful skill development. Playing a musical instrument similarly challenges several brain systems while providing an avenue for creative expression and potentially social connection through group music making. Complex hobbies such as chess, bridge, or crafting can provide ongoing cognitive challenges, while formal education at any age provides structured learning opportunities that maintain cognitive flexibility

Pillar 6: Stress Management: Protecting Your Cognitive Resources

Stress management is crucial for cognition. When stress hormones such as cortisol remain elevated over an extended period, they can damage memory centers, promote brain inflammation, and disrupt the neural networks that support executive function. The stress responses we explored in chapter 12—the fight-flight-freeze reactions that protect us from immediate danger—become problematic when chronically activated by ongoing life pressures.

Effective stress management for good cognitive health involves developing healthy responses to stress rather than attempting to eliminate stress entirely, which would be neither possible nor beneficial. Mindfulness practices, engaging in relaxation techniques regularly, time management strategies, and strong social support all help maintain the optimal arousal level that supports rather than impairs cognitive function.

Making Brain Health Sustainable: Start Small

Rather than overhauling your entire lifestyle at once, consider how small changes in each pillar can support your cognitive health ecosystem.

- **Exercise:** Add ten-minute walks to your existing routine before attempting hour-long gym sessions.
- **Nutrition:** Focus on adding brain-healthy foods to your diet rather than eliminating everything you enjoy.
- **Sleep:** Improve your sleep hygiene gradually; start with a consistent bedtime before addressing all sleep issues.
- **Social connection:** Prioritize quality over quantity; one meaningful conversation beats multiple superficial interactions.
- **Mental stimulation:** Choose challenges you genuinely enjoy rather than forcing yourself to go through tedious "brain training."
- **Stress management:** Find stress reduction techniques that fit your personality and schedule.

Remember: These pillars work synergistically. Improvements in one area often naturally support others. The same exercise that improves your sleep also enhances your mood and your energy for social connections.

Improving Your Brain: Evidence-Based Interventions

Beyond the foundational practices that support overall brain health, specific interventions can target particular aspects of cognitive function. These evidence-based approaches provide options for people who want to actively enhance their cognitive abilities rather than simply maintain their current function.

Mindfulness and meditation practices demonstrate increasingly robust scientific support for cognitive enhancement. Regular meditation produces measurable changes in brain structure and function, including increased gray matter volume in regions associated with attention and emotional regulation, improved connectivity among brain networks, enhanced attentional control and working memory, and reduced inflammation and stress hormone levels that can impair cognitive function.

Different forms of meditation support different cognitive domains. Focused attention practices, in which you concentrate on a single object such as your breath or a mantra, particularly strengthen sustained attention and concentration abilities. Open monitoring meditation, in which you observe your thoughts and sensations without getting caught up in them, enhances cognitive flexibility and metacognitive awareness—the ability to observe and understand your thinking processes.

The cognitive benefits of meditation don't require hours of daily practice or years of training to become apparent. Studies show meaningful improvements in attention and emotional regulation with practices as brief as ten to twenty minutes daily over several weeks. The key lies in consistency rather than duration, making meditation accessible even for people with busy schedules who might assume that they don't have time for this kind of cognitive training.

Targeted cognitive training can benefit specific cognitive functions when approached thoughtfully. While commercial "brain-training" programs make exaggerated claims about their effects transferring to general intelligence, carefully designed cognitive exercises can improve particular abilities when they sufficiently challenge your current capacity, adapt to performance improvements over time, transfer to real-world tasks, and are combined with other brain-healthy practices rather than serving as isolated interventions.

Rather than generic games or puzzles, effective cognitive training targets specific areas of concern or interest. Processing speed exercises might help people who feel that their thinking has slowed down, while working memory tasks can benefit those struggling with information management and complex task completion. Attention-training programs can help rebuild focusing capacity that has been compromised by chronic multitasking or high-stress environments.

As we discussed above, the most effective cognitive training occurs within the context of meaningful activities rather than abstract exercises. Learning new skills—languages, musical instruments, crafts, or games—trains and engages the brain much like weight-lifting improves muscle. The social element of activities such as playing bridge or singing in a choir provide an added brain boost.

Integration: Connecting Cognitive Health to Your Whole Health Ecosystem

The cognitive health strategies we've explored—exercise, nutrition, sleep optimization, attention training, social engagement, and stress management—are conscious interventions that you can implement deliberately. Yet their effectiveness often depends on unconscious factors that operate below the surface of awareness: the beliefs you hold about your cognitive capabilities, the automatic patterns that emerge under stress, and the narratives that determine whether you prioritize brain health or abandon these practices when life becomes challenging.

This interaction between conscious intention and unconscious patterns helps explain why cognitive health interventions sometimes succeed brilliantly while at other times fail despite our best conscious efforts. Someone might understand intellectually that exercise supports brain function but struggle to maintain consistent movement because unconscious beliefs about their body, aging, or worthiness of self-care undermine their conscious intentions. Another person might know that meditation enhances attention but find themselves unable to establish a regular practice because unconscious narratives about productivity and busyness make stillness feel like failure or a waste of time.

The attention difficulties and concentration problems discussed sometimes stem not from digital distraction or cognitive decline but from unconscious trauma responses. When past experiences create ongoing vigilance for danger, cognitive resources remain allocated to threat detection rather than available for focused thinking and memory consolidation. Understanding these deeper psychological dynamics often provides the missing piece for lasting cognitive health improvements.

Your cognitive health connects intimately with every other aspect of your health ecosystem. How you process and interpret health information—whether you catastrophize abnormal results or dismiss concerning symptoms—reflects cognitive patterns influenced by your attention, memory, and executive function. The choices you make about what to consume depend on your decision-making abilities, impulse control, and working memory capacity. Your ability to maintain consistent physical practices requires planning, organization, and the cognitive flexibility to adapt when circumstances change.

Understanding cognitive health as an integral part of your complete well-being helps explain why isolated interventions often fail while comprehensive approaches succeed. The exercise that protects your brain also supports your physical infrastructure. The nutrition that fuels your cognitive function also provides the energy for movement and cellular repair. The sleep that consolidates your memory also regulates the hormones that influence your mood, metabolism, and immune function.

The conscious efforts we make to support our cognitive health are only part of the story. Beneath our awareness lies a vast realm of unconscious processes, beliefs, and narratives that profoundly influence both our mental and physical health. Understanding this deeper layer of the mind completes our exploration of the INSIGHT quadrant.

14

The Unconscious Mind: The Stories We Tell Ourselves

Having explored the conscious dimensions of mental and cognitive health in chapters 12 and 13, we now turn to the unconscious mind, the hidden realm where core beliefs reside and "default settings" operate.

The unconscious mind is where you store your deepest assumptions about yourself, process emotions below the surface of consciousness, and automatically respond to life's challenges based on your past experiences and learned patterns. Your emotional responses, deeply ingrained habits, and automatic thoughts directly and profoundly influence every aspect of your physical health.

Understanding this unconscious realm—even acknowledging its existence and influence—is necessary for having genuine agency over your health.

The Iceberg of Consciousness

When I talk with patients about the unconscious mind, I often use the metaphor of an iceberg. What we see above the water—conscious thoughts, deliberate actions, and stated beliefs—represents only about 10 percent of our mental activity. The remaining 90 percent lies beneath the surface:

automatic responses, deeply held beliefs, emotional patterns, and narratives that we may not even realize are shaping our decisions.

This hidden terrain is where many of our health behaviors originate, where our relationships with food, exercise, medical care, and self-care are formed. When there's a disconnect between the conscious and unconscious parts of ourselves, we experience the all-too-familiar phenomenon of "knowing better but doing otherwise." We intellectually understand that we should eat nutritious foods, move our bodies regularly, and manage stress effectively—yet we find ourselves repeatedly making choices that undermine these goals.

The path toward greater health begins not with another diet plan or exercise regimen but with illuminating the iceberg, bringing the unconscious into our conscious awareness. This happens through curiosity, compassion, and a willingness to look beneath the surface of our behaviors.

The Stories We Tell Ourselves

Each of us carries a unique psychological blueprint that has been shaped by our life experiences, family dynamics, cultural context, and in some cases genetic tendencies toward certain emotional states or behavioral patterns. This blueprint influences how we respond to challenges, process information, and make health decisions. Whether we realize it or not, these patterns form the foundation of how we navigate the world and care for ourselves.

Some of your internal narratives may be true! Maybe you rose out of poverty, you were raised by an alcoholic parent, or you were bullied on the school bus as a child. But some parts of our internal narrative are not rooted in fact. These, too, inform our everyday health and decision-making. Sometimes these stories stem from childhood. Sometimes they result from an adverse experience. Sometimes they reflect a cultural reality, such as misogyny or racism, that we cannot easily change. The voices can be cruel, even punishing, when they tell us, for example, that we're unattractive, unfit, or unworthy of love. These narratives can directly inform our self-esteem, relationships, behaviors, and health, especially when we follow their script.

Consider, for example, my patient who convinced herself that she was not good enough. That narrative was born at a young age when she was teased in grade school for having difficulty learning to read. Her feelings of inadequacy were compounded by the absence of adequate support at home. By high school, she was depressed and binge eating. By college, she had developed a drinking problem and a full-blown eating disorder.

Adding to her problem is the fact that food manufacturers employ teams of food scientists to create products with precisely calibrated combinations of sugar, salt, fat, and flavor enhancers that maximize cravings and consumption. These formulations are tested and refined to ensure that they're "moreish"—that quality that makes you want to keep eating long after your hunger is satisfied. The phenomenon called "sensory-specific satiety" normally helps us stop eating when we've had enough of a particular food. However, processed foods with complex flavor profiles and textures can bypass this natural stopping mechanism, leading to what some researchers call "conditioned hypereating."

By the time I saw her as a new patient, she was on ten different medications, but no one in healthcare had ever asked her, "Tell me your story." Helping her wasn't just about diet and exercise; it involved unpacking the root cause of her emotional eating and self-soothing with food. This phenomenon is more common than people might think. We all do it on some level. It can be a result of growing up in a conflict-ridden, neglectful, or emotionally unavailable household. So for a patient with obesity and binge eating, the solution must begin with pulling the thread of an internal shame-based narrative. There's no diet for that.

The Inner Critic: Moving Beyond Self-Judgment

One of the most powerful unconscious narratives many of us carry involves harsh self-criticism that masquerades as motivation or self-improvement. While chapter 12 explored how societal stigma around mental health creates external barriers to care, the inner critic can interfere with health and well-being.

This inner voice is ever-present. It may comment on your food choices, judge your body size, or criticize your life choices. It may even provide a running commentary on your perceived inadequacies. Unlike the social stigma discussed earlier, the inner critic isn't about changing other people's minds about you; it demands integration of your unconscious and conscious worlds.

My patient Rebecca is a thirty-eight-year-old attorney and mother of two. She came to me complaining of persistent fatigue, frequent headaches, and digestive issues. Tests revealed mild inflammation but no clear disease process. As we talked, I noticed how often she disparaged herself: "I should be handling this better," "I'm being weak," "I can't believe I'm wasting your time with this." When I asked about her childhood, she revealed that she'd grown up with a father who had demanded perfection. Small mistakes meant harsh criticism; showing weakness was unacceptable. She'd internalized that voice so completely that she had pushed herself to the point of burnout—working sixty-hour weeks, exercising through pain, and denying herself basic needs such as sick days and adequate sleep.

Her physical symptoms weren't imaginary; they were very real manifestations of a body that had been denied permission to have limits. Her headaches often followed nights of insufficient sleep. Her digestive issues worsened during high-stress periods when she pushed the hardest. Her fatigue was the cumulative result of never allowing herself to rest until she collapsed.

Our work together focused not on silencing the inner critic—an impossible and perhaps undesirable goal—but on recognizing its voice, understanding its origins, and developing a more balanced internal dialogue. Rebecca began to notice the physical sensations that accompanied her self-criticism: tension in her shoulders, shallow breathing, a knot in her stomach. Those became cues to pause and ask, "Is this voice helping or harming me right now?"

Gradually she developed self-compassion, the ability to treat herself with the same loving-kindness she would offer a friend in similar circumstances. When she made a mistake, she learned to acknowledge it without defining herself by it. When she needed rest, she began to honor that need rather than pushing through. The change in her physical health was remarkable. Her headaches decreased in frequency and severity. Her digestive symptoms improved. Her energy level became more consistent. Most important, she developed what I call "sustainable health behaviors": practices she could maintain without the exhausting cycle of perfectionism and burnout that had characterized her previous approach.

People Pleasing: When Others' Needs Override Your Own

Another common narrative I see in my practice centers on the belief "My needs don't matter as much as others'." This belief often manifests itself as people-pleasing behavior: prioritizing others' needs, opinions, and comfort above one's own, sometimes to the point of losing touch with one's own personal desires and boundaries.

Jerome, a fifty-two-year-old teacher, came to see me with what he described as "stress-related problems": high blood pressure, insomnia, and recurrent chest pain that cardiac workups had deemed to be noncardiac. As we explored his daily routines, I noticed a pattern: Jerome never said no. To anyone. He volunteered for extra committees at school. He was the family member everyone called in a crisis. He spent weekends helping friends with home repairs and evenings counseling colleagues through their personal problems. When I asked about his own needs, he looked genuinely confused. "I don't really think about that," he admitted. Further conversation revealed a childhood in which his emotional needs had consistently been ignored while he was praised for being "helpful" and "not causing trouble." He'd learned that his value came from serving others, not from his inherent worth as a person.

That narrative had had direct health consequences. He routinely sacrificed sleep to help others. He skipped meals when someone needed his attention. He ignored the early warning signs of burnout because addressing them would mean setting boundaries—something his internal narrative classified as "selfish."

Jerome needed to be reconnected with his own needs and desires—a process that felt foreign and even frightening at first. We started small: identifying one personal preference each day, scheduling nonnegotiable time for basic self-care, practicing saying "I need to think about it" before saying yes to requests. The most transformative moment came when he realized that his people pleasing wasn't serving others as well as he'd thought. His resentment had been building. His effectiveness had been diminishing as his health deteriorated. The quality of his relationships had been suffering because they lacked authenticity.

As he learned to honor his own needs alongside others', his blood pressure stabilized. His sleep improved. The episodes of chest pain became less frequent. Most important, he discovered that setting healthy boundaries didn't destroy his relationships; it transformed them into more genuine connections based on mutual respect rather than caretaking and dependence. Jerome's experience illustrates how unconscious narratives affect every aspect of the health ecosystem; his people-pleasing patterns had influenced not only his cardiovascular health and sleep quality (INFRASTRUCTURE impacts) but also his eating patterns as he skipped meals to help others (INPUTS effects) and his ability to accurately assess and communicate his own health status to medical providers (INFORMATICS complications).

Perfectionism: The Myth of Always Being "Just Right"

Our culture's emphasis on perfection—in appearance, achievement, and behavior—creates another powerful narrative that affects our health in profound ways. The belief that we must appear perfect to be worthy often leads to a split between our public persona and our private reality, creating immense psychological strain and undermining authentic self-care.

Linda, a forty-five-year-old marketing executive, maintained an impeccable image: successful career, beautiful home, active in community causes, always well dressed and composed. She came to me with vague complaints: fatigue, minor aches and pains, nothing that showed up on standard tests. What was most striking was her insistence that apart from those minor issues, everything was "perfect."

Only after several visits did the facade begin to crack. She revealed that she was drinking a bottle of wine most nights to manage anxiety. Her marriage was deeply troubled. She was having panic attacks in private but maintaining her composed exterior at all costs. The narrative driving this behavior was clear: "If people saw the real me, with all my flaws and struggles, I would lose everything."

This gulf between public perfection and private suffering created constant vigilance—an exhausting state that manifested itself in physical symptoms. The effort to maintain her "perfect person" image had prevented her from seeking appropriate help for her anxiety and alcohol use. It had kept her isolated in her marital problems. It had made authentic self-care impossible, as any acknowledgment of need threatened the perfection narrative.

Linda needed to acknowledge her challenges without shame and seek support without feeling diminished. Doing so wasn't easy; the perfect-person narrative had served important protective functions throughout her life. But as she began taking small risks—sharing her struggles with trusted friends, addressing issues in therapy rather than self-medicating, prioritizing genuine well-being over appearance—her physical symptoms began to resolve. The fatigue lifted as she reduced her alcohol intake and addressed her anxiety more effectively. The diffuse pain diminished as the constant tension of vigilance eased. Most important, she began experiencing what many of my patients describe as "relief": the profound unburdening that comes from living more authentically, from no longer having to maintain the exhausting split between public persona and private reality.

The Trauma Response: When the Past Dictates the Present

Some of the most powerful narratives affecting our health stem from traumatic experiences. These events create both explicit stories we tell ourselves ("The world isn't safe") and body responses that bypass conscious thought entirely. Understanding how trauma shapes our health—often beneath our conscious awareness—is essential for true healing.

Marty, a thirty-five-year-old programmer, came to me with irritable bowel syndrome that had persisted despite dietary changes and medications. During our conversations, he mentioned a car accident he'd experienced as a teenager. While he hadn't been seriously injured, the accident had been terrifying, leaving him trapped in the vehicle for nearly an hour before help had arrived. What he hadn't understood was how his body still carried that experience. His digestive symptoms often worsened when he felt trapped or helpless—in traffic jams, crowded elevators, or high-pressure work situations. His body was responding to those triggers as if the original danger were present, activating the fight-flight-freeze response that directly affects gut function.

The narrative Marty had developed wasn't explicit but operated powerfully beneath the surface: "When I'm not in complete control, disaster follows." That had led to hypervigilance, muscle tension, and activation of stress responses in situations that resembled aspects of the original trauma, often without his conscious awareness. Our approach to his healing involved both somatic (body-based) and cognitive work. Marty learned to recognize the physical sensations that signaled that his trauma response was activating. He developed techniques to ground himself in the present moment, distinguishing between past danger and present safety. He began to create a new narrative that acknowledged his experience while recognizing his current resources and agency.

As Marty's nervous system began to regulate itself more effectively, his digestive symptoms improved dramatically. The connection between his past trauma and his present physical distress became clearer, allowing for more targeted interventions. Most important, he gained a compassionate understanding of his symptoms, not as something wrong with him but as his body's attempt to protect him based on his past experience.

The stories of Rebecca, James, Linda, and Marty illustrate how our unconscious narratives, whether rooted in perfectionism, people pleasing, facade maintenance, or trauma responses, create very real physical symptoms and health challenges. While each person's unconscious patterns were unique, they all shared a common experience: Their bodies were responding to beliefs and emotional patterns operating below their conscious awareness. Recognizing these patterns in yourself requires a different kind of data collection than tracking steps or monitoring blood pressure does. It involves developing the capacity to observe your internal landscape with curiosity rather than judgment, to notice the subtle connections among thoughts, emotions, and physical sensations that reveal the unconscious forces that shape your health behaviors.

Collecting Data About Your Unconscious Mind

How can you begin illuminating these unconscious narratives? It starts with data collection—not spreadsheets or fitness tracker metrics but a different kind of information gathering. It's about learning to observe without judgment, to notice patterns in our reactions, and to approach yourself with curiosity rather than criticism.

In my practice, I encourage patients to ask themselves:

- What situations consistently trigger strong emotional reactions?
- What phrases do I repeatedly tell myself?
- What physical sensations accompany difficult emotions?

- When do my health symptoms tend to worsen or improve?
- What patterns emerge in my relationships with others?

This isn't about analyzing every thought or feeling—an impossible and potentially counterproductive task; it's about developing what mindfulness traditions call the "observing self," the part of you that can step back and notice patterns without being completely identified with them.

One simple but powerful practice involves keeping a journal in which you record situations that trigger strong emotions, the thoughts that accompany those emotions, and the behaviors that follow. Over time, patterns typically emerge; the same core beliefs appear in different contexts, the same reactions occur to similar triggers. These patterns provide invaluable clues to the unconscious narratives shaping your health behaviors. The perfectionist who skips meals when work gets busy; the people pleaser who neglects sleep to meet others' needs; the trauma survivor whose symptoms flare in situations resembling past threats; in all these cases, with awareness comes the possibility of choice—not immediate control but the beginning of a different relationship with these patterns.

Fact-Checking Your Internal Narrative

Once you've identified potential narratives, the next essential step is to fact-check them against reality. This isn't about positive thinking or forced optimism; it's about developing a more accurate understanding of yourself and your experiences.

The process begins with questions such as:

- Is this belief always true, or are there exceptions?
- Where did I learn this narrative? Is the source reliable?
- What evidence supports or contradicts this belief?
- How would I view this situation if it were happening to someone else?
- What other perspectives might be equally or more accurate?

This fact-checking process isn't a onetime event but an ongoing practice of bringing conscious awareness to your unconscious assumptions. It's about developing what psychologists call "cognitive flexibility," the ability to consider multiple perspectives rather than being locked into rigid patterns of thought.

I often suggest that patients experiment with alternative narratives—not forcing themselves to believe something new but simply trying on different perspectives to see how they fit. "What if my worth isn't determined by my productivity?" "What if some of my physical symptoms are related to emotions I haven't processed?" "What if asking for help is a sign of strength rather than weakness?" These experiments create space between stimulus and response—a pause in which new possibilities can emerge. They don't erase established neural pathways overnight, but they begin laying down alternative routes that can, with practice, become more accessible.

The Path Toward Integration: Finding Your Wise Mind

In dialectical behavior therapy (DBT), there's a concept called "wise mind"—the integration of emotional mind (feelings, intuition, desires) and reasonable mind (logic, facts, analysis). This integrated state represents a balance in which both emotion and reason inform your choices, where you can acknowledge your feelings without being controlled by them. But this practice can also have very tangible results on your physical health and biomarkers. Despite being considered "woo woo" by traditional medicine, developing personal insight directly impacts medical INFORMATICS. Developing wise mind is a gradual process that involves four key practices.

Mindfulness: The Science of Present-Moment Awareness

Research in neuroscience has demonstrated that regular mindfulness practice creates measurable changes in brain structure and function. Studies using functional MRI (fMRI) have shown that mindfulness strengthens the connections between the prefrontal cortex (responsible for executive function) and the amygdala (our threat detection center), allowing for better emotional regulation. In 2018, a meta-analysis published in *JAMA Internal Medicine* found that mindfulness meditation helps reduce chronic pain intensity by 30 percent in some patients—equivalent to some prescription medications but without side effects. Additionally, mindfulness practices have been shown to reduce inflammatory markers such as C-reactive protein and interleukin-6, which are associated with numerous chronic diseases.

Iman, a forty-two-year-old accountant, came to me with chronic tension headaches and jaw pain from temporomandibular joint (TMJ) disorder. Traditional treatments had provided only temporary relief. Through our work together, Iman began practicing mindfulness daily, learning to scan her body for early signs of tension. She noticed that she routinely clenched her jaw during stressful work calls and when reading certain emails. By developing the ability to notice this tension without judgment, she could consciously relax those muscles before the tension escalated to pain. Within two months, her headache frequency decreased by over 50 percent, and her need for pain medication diminished significantly. The pain hadn't disappeared completely, but her relationship with it had transformed; it was no longer something that controlled her day.

Self-Compassion: The Science of Kind Self-Regard

Research by Dr. Kristin Neff and others has demonstrated that self-compassion—treating oneself with kindness rather than harsh criticism—produces significant physiological benefits. Self-compassion practices reduce cortisol (the stress hormone) and increase heart rate variability (a marker of cardiovascular health and stress resilience). In 2021, a study published in *Health Psychology* showed that individuals with higher self-compassion had lower inflammatory responses to stress and faster recovery times after illness. Additionally, self-compassion appears to mitigate the negative health effects of perfectionism, which has been linked to insomnia, compromised immune function, and increased cardiovascular risk.

Stewart, a fifty-six-year-old executive, had struggled with hypertension for years despite medication and conventional lifestyle advice. His self-talk was relentlessly critical: Every dietary slip became evidence of "weakness," every missed workout proof of "laziness." That harsh inner dialogue triggered stress responses that directly affected his blood pressure. We worked on his developing self-compassion practices, including a brief daily meditation during which he offered himself the same kindness that he would show a friend facing similar challenges. His blood pressure readings gradually stabilized as he replaced self-criticism with self-support. More surprisingly, his adherence to his health regimen improved with this gentler approach; he found it easier to maintain healthy behaviors when they weren't driven by fear and self-punishment.

Dialectical Thinking: The Science of Holding Complexity

Cognitive flexibility, the ability to accept different concepts or perspectives rather than take an all-or-nothing approach, has been linked to resilience and better health outcomes. Research at Columbia University has demonstrated that individuals who can hold seemingly contradictory truths simultaneously (a key aspect of dialectical thinking) demonstrate greater immune function and recover more quickly from inflammatory conditions—they experience less of the physiological "wear and tear" that chronic stress places on the body.

Bina, a thirty-eight-year-old teacher with autoimmune thyroiditis, initially approached her condition with rigid black-and-white thinking. She oscillated between perfect adherence to her treatment plan and complete abandonment of it when she couldn't maintain ideal standards. That all-or-nothing approach kept her health unstable and her symptoms flaring. Through our work together, she developed dialectical thinking, the ability to hold the idea that she could be both sick and well, that she could accept her condition while working to improve it, that some days would be better than others without defining her entire journey. As she embraced that more nuanced perspective, her symptom management improved markedly. Her thyroid antibodies, a marker of autoimmune activity, decreased by 40 percent over six months. Equally important, her quality of life improved as she moved away from the exhausting pendulum of perfectionism and resignation.

Emotional Regulation: The Science of Feeling Without Becoming Overwhelmed

Emotional regulation directly impacts physical health through multiple pathways. Research has shown that poor emotional regulation is associated with increased inflammation, compromised immune function, and higher rates of cardiovascular disease. Conversely, effective emotional regulation skills have been linked to lower blood pressure, improved glycemic control in diabetes, and reduced symptoms in chronic pain conditions. A groundbreaking study at the University of Wisconsin demonstrated that individuals trained in emotional regulation techniques showed increased activity in genes that counter inflammation and decreased activity in pro-inflammatory genes after just eight weeks.

Arthur, a forty-five-year-old software engineer with IBS, had tried several dietary approaches with limited success. Through careful tracking, we discovered that his symptoms spiked not just when he consumed certain foods but in response to specific emotional states—particularly suppressed anger and anxiety. He learned emotion regulation techniques, including identifying his emotions earlier, naming them, and responding skillfully rather than suppressing or overreacting. He created a "feelings wheel" on his phone to help precisely identify what he was experiencing and corresponding strategies for each emotion. Within three months, his IBS symptoms had improved by approximately 60 percent. Laboratory tests showed reduced inflammatory markers, and his microbiome diversity—a measure of gut health—had improved significantly. Arthur noted that the skills he had learned transferred to other areas of his life as well, improving his sleep quality and reducing the tension headaches that had previously been a weekly occurrence.

When the Inner World Stays Hidden: The Cost of Denial and the Freedom of Truth Telling

Many patients resist looking within. They avoid regular check-ins with themselves or their doctor. They may diligently monitor certain aspects of their health while ignoring others. They usually say that they don't have time, they're too busy, or they've always been healthy and expect problems to resolve on their own. This avoidance reflects what psychologists call *denial*, a defense mechanism that protects us from dealing with painful truths we're not yet ready to face. While denial can provide temporary emotional shelter, it ultimately extracts a steep cost from our health and well-being.

As the saying goes, "The truth will set you free, but first it will make you miserable." This insight, often attributed to President James A. Garfield but echoing biblical wisdom from John 8:32 ("You will know the truth, and the truth will set you free"), captures the paradoxical nature of confronting difficult realities. There is indeed emotional pain in recognizing patterns we've long denied, but this temporary discomfort paves the way for authentic healing that denial cannot provide.

The Cost of Denial

Recent research on the ways in which our psychology affects our nervous and immune systems has demonstrated that denial isn't just psychologically taxing; it creates measurable physiological stress.

A study published in the *Journal of Behavioral Medicine* in 2019 found that emotional suppression and avoidance were associated with increased inflammatory markers, particularly interleukin-6 and C-reactive protein, both linked to chronic disease development. Brain-imaging studies have shown that denial requires constant unconscious monitoring of the denied material, consuming neural resources that could otherwise support healing and growth. In other words, what we resist *persists*, not just in our minds but in our bodies. The energy required to maintain denial depletes the resources needed for immune function, tissue repair, and other essential physiological processes. Allison, a fifty-seven-year-old teacher with two years of severe migraines and fatigue, had seen multiple specialists without improvement. What she hadn't mentioned was that her symptoms had begun after her mother's death, for which she had taken only three days off work. "That's all behind me now," she said dismissively.

Her body told a different story through her elevated cortisol level and inflammatory markers. After we built trust, Allison began working with a grief counselor to process her complicated relationship with her mother. Her migraine frequency decreased by 70 percent, her sleep improved, and her stress markers normalized. "I thought I was being strong by not dealing with my grief," she reflected. "Instead, I was just forcing my body to carry what my mind wouldn't acknowledge."

The Courage to Look Within

Breaking through denial requires courage and the willingness to increase discomfort temporarily for the sake of long-term healing. It often requires support as well, whether from healthcare providers, therapists, trusted friends, or support groups. Few of us can face difficult truths entirely alone.

For those contemplating this journey, I offer these guidelines.

- **Start with self-compassion.** Approach self-discovery with kindness rather than judgment. Denial doesn't develop because we're weak or flawed; it emerges as a protective mechanism in response to pain we weren't equipped to process at the time.
- **Seek appropriate support.** Different situations require different types of support. Addiction may require specialized treatment; grief might benefit from counseling; relationship issues might call for couples therapy. Don't try to do this work alone if you don't have to.

- **Move at a sustainable pace.** Breaking through denial doesn't have to happen all at once. Even small acknowledgments of previously avoided truths can begin shifting physiological patterns in positive directions.
- **Recognize the physical benefits.** Pay attention to how your body responds as you begin to acknowledge difficult realities. Many patients report improved sleep, decreased pain, better digestion, and more stable energy levels—concrete evidence that the truth truly does set us free both physically and emotionally.

Red Flags: When to Seek Professional Help with Unconscious Patterns

While self-exploration and awareness can powerfully transform health outcomes, some situations require professional support. Consider seeking help from a therapist, counselor, or other mental health professional when the following situations exist.

Immediate Safety Concerns

- Thoughts of self-harm or suicide
- Substance use that feels out of control or dangerous
- Eating behaviors that significantly impact your physical health
- Relationship patterns involving abuse or violence

Persistent Patterns Despite Awareness

- You recognize unhealthy patterns but feel unable to change them despite sustained effort.
- Your physical symptoms worsen or don't improve even as you address unconscious factors.
- The same destructive cycles repeat in your relationship, work, or health behaviors.
- Your self-criticism becomes so harsh that it interferes with your daily functioning.

Trauma-Related Responses

- Physical symptoms that seem connected to past traumatic experiences
- Panic attacks, flashbacks, or dissociative episodes
- Hypervigilance or feeling constantly unsafe without an obvious current threat
- Avoidance behaviors that significantly limit your life activities

When Self-Exploration Feels Overwhelming

- Uncovering unconscious patterns triggers intense emotional reactions that you can't manage alone.
- You feel stuck in analysis without being able to move toward healing.
- Your family or relationship dynamics make individual change feel impossible.
- Your past experiences feel too painful or complex to process without support.

Professional Support Options

- **Therapists/counselors:** For individual therapy focusing on unconscious patterns and health behaviors
- **Trauma specialists:** For eye movement desensitization and reprocessing (EMDR), somatic therapy, or other trauma-informed approaches
- **Psychiatrists:** For medication evaluation when your mental health significantly impacts your physical health
- **Health psychologists:** For specialists who understand mind-body connections in medical settings
- **Support groups:** For peer support around specific issues such as grief, addiction, and chronic illness

How to Find Quality Care

- Ask your primary care provider for referrals to mental health professionals.
- Check with your insurance company for covered providers.
- Look for therapists with experience in health psychology or medical issues.

- Consider whether you need someone who specializes in your specific concerns (trauma, eating disorders, addiction, etc.).
- Don't hesitate to interview potential therapists to find a good fit.

Remember: Seeking professional help isn't a sign of weakness or failure; it's a wise recognition that some unconscious patterns developed in response to experiences that require specialized support to heal. Just as you wouldn't try to treat a broken bone without medical help, some psychological wounds need professional intervention to heal properly.

The goal is integration and healing that supports your complete health ecosystem, not endless analysis or dependence on therapy. A skilled professional will help you develop the tools and insights you need to continue your growth independently.

KNOW YOURSELF, ADVOCATE FOR YOURSELF

Your INSIGHT Reflection and Action Guide

PART 1 Self-Reflection: Understanding Your INSIGHT Quadrant

Pull out your pen and paper again! This final quadrant—your mental, cognitive, and emotional health—ties everything else together.

Your Mental and Emotional Health

- How would you describe your baseline emotional state? Anxious? Content? Resilient? Overwhelmed?
- When stress hits, how far do you "travel" from your baseline? Do you bounce back quickly or stay elevated for days?
- What mental health challenges have you experienced—anxiety, depression, grief, trauma? How have these affected your physical health?
- How honest are you with yourself (and others) about your mental health struggles?
- What tools do you currently use to manage stress, loss, and uncertainty? Are they working?
- Who in your life actually sees and supports your mental health? Who could you talk to more openly?
- If you approached your health with compassion rather than judgment, what would change?

Your Cognitive Health

- What are your cognitive strengths? Sharp memory? Good problem-solver? Quick with words?
- What cognitive challenges do you notice? Trouble focusing? Forgetting things? Brain fog?
- Have you noticed changes in your thinking, memory, or attention over time? When did you first notice them?

- What environments or activities make your brain work best? Worst?
- How honest are you being about any cognitive struggles you're experiencing?

The Stories You Tell Yourself (Your Unconscious Mind)

- What situations consistently trigger strong emotional reactions in you? (Notice the pattern, not just the individual moments.)
- What does your inner critic tell you? "I'm not good enough," "I have to be perfect," "I can't trust my body," "Showing weakness is dangerous"?
- What physical sensations come up when you're emotionally distressed? Tight chest? Stomach knots? Tension headaches?
- When do your health symptoms tend to flare up? During conflict? After saying yes when you meant no? When you're overwhelmed at work?
- What health behaviors do you "know better" about but keep doing anyway?
- Looking at your relationships—with food, with your body, with exercise, with doctors—what patterns show up repeatedly?
- If your symptoms could talk, what would they be trying to tell you about your life?
- What beliefs about yourself might be driving unhealthy behaviors? (Example: "I don't deserve care" → skipping doctor appointments; "I must never fail" → pushing through injury.)
- Where did you learn these patterns? Childhood? Past trauma? Cultural messages? Family dynamics?
- What parts of your health and life are you avoiding looking at?

Connections Across Your Health

- How does stress or anxiety affect what and when you eat, drink, and consume?
- How does your mental state influence your energy for movement and exercise?
- How do your thoughts and emotions show up as physical symptoms in your body?
- How does your cognitive function impact your ability to interpret medical information, weigh risks and benefits, and make health decisions?

Reclaiming Agency

- Where do you feel you have real control over your mental and cognitive health?
- Where do you feel stuck or powerless?
- What's one small, specific action you could take this week to support your mental health?
- If you could fact-check one belief you hold about yourself, which would you choose?
- What might be possible if you brought more awareness to the unconscious patterns driving your health behaviors?

PART 2 Healthcare Conversations: Questions and Strategies for Medical Encounters

Questions to Ask Your Medical Provider

- "What is one small, specific action I could take this week to start improving my mental and/or cognitive health?"
- "How might stress or emotional factors be affecting my physical symptoms?"
- "Could my [sleep problems/mood changes/chronic pain] be related to my cognitive concerns?"
- "I've noticed changes in my [memory/attention/thinking]. What evaluation would you recommend?"
- "How can I tell the difference between normal aging and cognitive changes that need evaluation?"
- "Are any of my current medications associated with cognitive or mood side effects?"
- "What mental health resources would you recommend for someone with my situation?"
- "How can I distinguish between physical symptoms and anxiety-related symptoms?"
- "What approaches have helped your other patients cope with this diagnosis?"

- "Based on my health history and risk factors, what should I be doing now to protect my brain health?"

Communication Strategies

- Share relevant emotional experiences without minimizing your physical symptoms.
- Be specific about what you're experiencing: "I can't focus for more than ten minutes" is more helpful than "My brain feels foggy."
- Articulate patterns you've noticed: "My symptoms get worse when I'm stressed" or "I sleep better when I exercise."
- Ask about mind-body connections specific to your condition.
- Request screening for mental and cognitive health issues when appropriate—don't wait to be asked.
- Discuss how to address both physical and emotional aspects of your health issues together.
- Explain what barriers may prevent you from prioritizing your mental health (time, money, stigma, not knowing where to start).
- Express your desire for additional support to maintain or improve your mental and cognitive well-being.
- Ask for specific ways you can measure progress beyond just "feeling better."

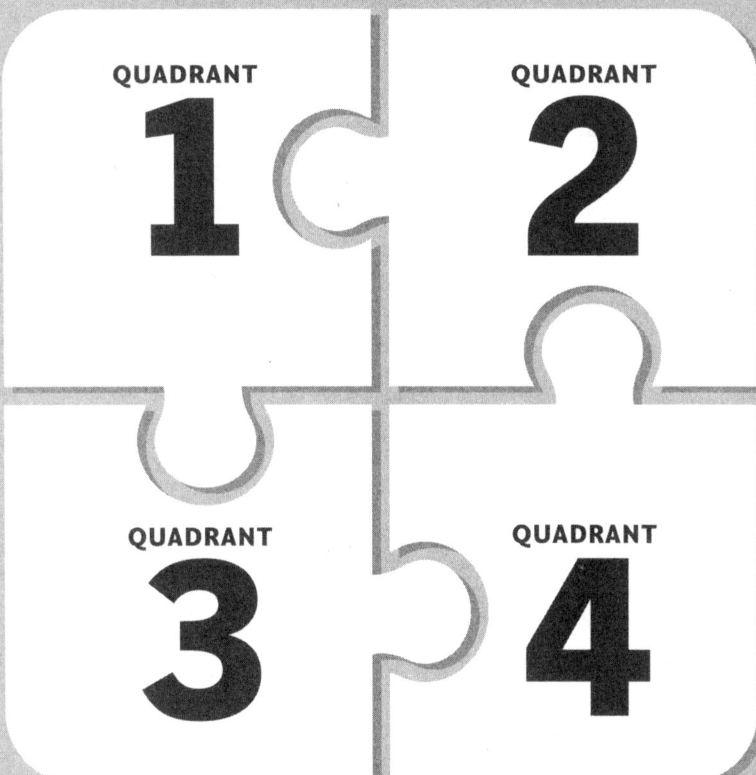

PUTTING IT ALL TOGETHER

You've now explored the complete landscape of your health ecosystem. You understand that your INFORMATICS quadrant captures both the medical data doctors measure and the biographic data that shapes your health story. You've examined your INPUTS—what you eat, drink, and ingest—and how these choices ripple through your entire system. You've assessed your INFRASTRUCTURE, recognizing that movement, physical capability, and the structural support of your body form the foundation for daily function. And you've delved into INSIGHT, discovering how mental health, cognitive function, and the unconscious stories you tell yourself influence every aspect of your well-being.

The four quadrants provide a map. But a map alone doesn't get you where you need to go. The next section focuses on you—the navigator of your own health journey. Here, we shift from understanding your ecosystem to actively engaging with it.

Owning Your Role in Your Own Healthcare

Now that you've redefined health on your terms and mapped your health ecosystem, your next steps are about putting your knowledge into action. This is where you learn to translate knowledge into action, where self-awareness becomes self-advocacy, and where you discover how to work effectively within (and sometimes around) our imperfect healthcare system. It's about recognizing your patient personality, asking for the right help at the right time, and practicing acceptance of what cannot be changed while focusing your energy on what you can influence. In today's hurried healthcare settings, self-advocacy is essential. It's not just about speaking up; it's about understanding what version of yourself shows up at the doctor's office, leveraging your interpersonal skills, recognizing how you get in your own way, and having realistic expectations for yourself and those who care for you. Let's walk through these final three steps now.

Step 3: Understand Your Patient Personality

Each of us brings a unique version of ourselves to every medical encounter, what I call our "patient personality": our set of biases, mental shortcuts, and belief systems that inform how we ask for and accept medical help. Your patient personality reflects how you make sense of medical information, what you reveal about yourself to your doctors, and how you approach making medical decisions.

For example, when experiencing chest discomfort, an **Optimizer** might first try doing breathing exercises, a **Pleaser** would downplay symptoms to avoid bothering the doctor, an **Internet Warrior** would research heart attack symptoms and seek "natural" solutions online, and an **Outsourcer** would want a doctor's appointment right away and know where to pick up a prescription.

Your patient personality may not reflect your true personality. In addition, it may change over time. After a cancer diagnosis, for example, I have witnessed some patients abandon a posture of stoicism and engage more with their healthcare team. I have seen other patients shed their doctor-pleasing tendencies and become better self-advocates over time. You may recognize yourself in one or more of these archetypes. You may be a Venn diagram of two or more overlapping personality types.

Regardless of where you fit in, understanding your patient personality isn't about labels or judgment. It's also not about blaming the victim of our wonky system! It's about cultivating self-awareness as the first step toward self-advocacy. It's about recognizing how healthcare providers may perceive you. Getting smart about your biases, beliefs, and communication style can help you work more efficiently with providers and get the care you need.

Each patient personality type has strengths and limitations that can impact your interactions with healthcare professionals. For example, your thorough internet research in advance of medical appointments may lead to more personalized care and better-informed decisions; it may also set you up for heightened anxiety, difficulty making decisions, or reluctance to accept medical advice.

Understanding this duality is crucial because no patient personality is inherently "good" or "bad"; each is a natural response to vulnerability. But when you start to recognize your patterns of engagement with medical providers, you can leverage your natural strengths and be aware of barriers that may be preventing you from getting what you need. You might try communicating your style to your healthcare providers to improve your care. A simple statement such as "I tend to minimize my symptoms, so I've written everything down" or "I'm a natural skeptic, so I will have lots of questions" or "My health anxiety is not about you; it's a result of bad experiences in the past" gives your provider valuable context for tailoring their approach. It also helps buttress your relationship. Transparency creates room for genuine collaboration rather than the frustrating dance of mismatched expectations that characterizes so many medical interactions.

Patient Personality Pop Quiz: Which Sounds Most Like You?

Before we dive deeper, consider which of these statements resonates most strongly with you:

- "I believe I can optimize my health through discipline, research, and the right lifestyle choices." (the **Optimizer**)
- "I rarely question my doctor's recommendations. They're the expert, after all." Or "It's important to me to maintain a positive relationship with my doctor, even when I don't necessarily agree with everything they say." (the **Pleaser**)
- "When something feels wrong, I immediately research it online to understand what might be happening." (the **Internet Warrior**)
- "Medical decisions should be left to the experts. I just want solutions." (the **Outsourcer**)

Most people identify with elements of several types but usually have one or two dominant patterns. Recognizing yours can transform how you approach healthcare and the patient-doctor relationship.

The Optimizer

Core belief: "I can control my health through discipline, research, and the right lifestyle choices."

This is the person who believes in using willpower to manage and solve most health problems. They like rules and crave certainty. They tend to have an outsized sense of control over their health and life. Doctors love Optimizers! They are often diligent exercisers. They are typically high achievers, even perfectionists. They listen to and follow longevity influencers such as Peter Attia and Andrew Huberman. They love tracking their steps, grams of protein, and sleep. They make conscious efforts to limit their caffeine, alcohol, and sugar intake—that is, until they fall off the wagon and beat themselves up for it.

Optimizers struggle with gray areas. Navigating the space between "ideal" and sustainable health behaviors causes them distress. As a result, they often adopt rigid health routines to avoid the gray areas altogether. But when life gets messy or emotions flare, their relative inflexibility makes navigating uncertainty more difficult. When an Optimizer falls short, they engage in self-soothing behaviors and feel guilty the next day.

Of course, striving to be healthy is good! The problem is that willpower and personal optimization aren't sufficient for health. Take Steve, a fit fifty-four-year-old who always arrived at my office with a spreadsheet tracking his exercise, sleep, and nutrition. He managed his stress with cold-water plunges. He believed that his normal weight and regular fitness routine meant he was completely healthy, but his family history revealed a strong risk of developing coronary artery disease. His lab tests showed a very high lipoprotein(a) level, indicating an increased risk of heart attack and stroke. I suggested that he undergo a coronary artery calcium scan to check for plaque buildup. "I seriously doubt I have heart disease," he responded. "I just ran a half-marathon." After two years of persistently abnormal test results, he finally agreed. The scan revealed significant plaque buildup in his coronary arteries, despite his excellent fitness level. He beat himself up about that finding, even though it had nothing to do with his habits. I told him that he needed to keep up his excellent habits; he also needed to treat a serious medical condition and to give himself permission to be human.

Working with Your Optimizer Tendencies

- **Strengths to leverage:** Your commitment to healthy habits and personal responsibility over your health is commendable.
- **Watch for blind spots:** Remember that perfect habits don't guarantee perfect outcomes. Health is an interplay of genetics, lifestyle, environment, and sometimes bad luck.
- **Growth opportunities:** Ask yourself if your habits are masking unmet social-emotional needs. Work on accepting what you cannot control while continuing to optimize what you can. Consider how medical interventions might complement rather than replace your lifestyle approach.

The Pleaser

Core belief: "Good patients follow instructions, are agreeable, and don't waste their doctor's time."

The Pleaser approaches healthcare with a profound desire for external validation. They tend to outsource their intuition and measure their worth through others' opinions and judgments. They would rather "win" the appointment with their doctor than worry their doctor about their symptoms. They often display "white coat worship," deferring to medical authority figures and rarely questioning recommendations or expressing concerns, even when those concerns could be critical to their care. Pleasers frequently minimize symptoms until they become unmanageable, fearing that they'll be seen as difficult and demanding. Pleasers' disconnect from their own wisdom runs deeper than simple courtesy or respect for expertise; it represents a fundamental diminishment of self in medical contexts.

Susie, a seventy-year-old active woman with impeccable manners, arrived at my office with a walking boot on her right foot, the result of her third fracture in four months. During our appointment, she struggled to describe her falling episodes, prefacing each description with a qualifier: "It's probably just my clumsiness" or "I don't want to make a fuss." When I asked how the falls had impacted her daily life and travel plans, she hesitated before saying "It's just a minor inconvenience," even though her medical record documented several emergency room visits and significant injuries.

I discovered that the ER physician had recommended that she use a cane for stability, which Susie confirmed she was using. Only later did she reluctantly admit that she felt self-conscious about using a mobility aid in public and mostly left it at home. "My father was a doctor," she explained. "I have tremendous respect for the medical profession and wouldn't want to disappoint him or you." I gently explained to her that she needed to have a bone density scan, a consultation with a neurologist, and a home safety evaluation. More important, she needed to practice making her needs known.

Working with Your Pleaser Tendencies

- **Strengths to leverage:** Your respect for expertise and commitment to following doctors' advice can lead to positive health outcomes and promote productive partnerships in healthcare.
- **Watch for blind spots:** The focus on people pleasing can interfere with getting your needs met. Withholding your concerns or symptoms can lead to missed diagnoses and suboptimal care.
- **Growth opportunities:** Practice being honest about your needs and giving yourself permission to have them. Prepare questions before appointments and speak up when something doesn't feel right. Remember that the patient-doctor relationship requires honesty and truth first.

The Internet Warrior

Core belief: "I need to research extensively to understand what's happening with my body."

The Internet Warrior participates actively in their healthcare, but they are easily misled by online health information. They tend to distrust doctors, favoring self-diagnosis by doing their own research or using symptom checkers such as ChatGPT. They are drawn to holistic, nonpharmaceutical interventions, often viewing them as safer alternatives to conventional treatments. They research extensively about natural remedies, lifestyle medicine, and alternative health paradigms. They desire control but become overwhelmed with the vast amount of online information—which only fuels more research. They often value the body's innate healing capacity but may sometimes delay necessary conventional treatments while exploring alternatives. Their vigilance often provides them comfort, an unconscious shield against vulnerability.

Emma, a sixty-two-year-old retired teacher, had always been proactive about her health. With a history of mild hypothyroidism, occasional migraines, and chronic lower back pain, she knew how to manage her conditions. But when she started experiencing new symptoms—fatigue and tingling in her hands—her usual sense of control unraveled. She started with reputable medical websites but soon found herself in forums where personal anecdotes about devastating neurological conditions dominated. Her anxiety grew with each search, creating a feedback loop in which her symptoms worsened, prompting more desperate research.

By the time she came to see me, she'd convinced herself that she had MS, ALS, or early-onset dementia. The anxiety itself was creating physical symptoms: disrupted sleep, muscle tension, hyperawareness of normal sensations. What she needed wasn't more information but help with medical context and tools to manage her internet-fueled anxiety.

Working with Your Internet Warrior Tendencies

- **Strengths to leverage:** Your engagement with your health and desire to understand medical conditions can make you an informed, active participant in your care.
- **Watch for blind spots:** Online information lacks clinical context and doesn't account for your specific medical history. Self-diagnosis based on internet research often focuses on worst-case scenarios rather than statistical probabilities.
- **Growth opportunities:** Set boundaries around your medical research. Limit your time spent researching symptoms, stick to reputable sources, and save questions for healthcare providers rather than seeking answers exclusively online.

The Outsourcer

Core belief: "Medical decisions should be left to the experts. I just want solutions."

The Outsourcer tends to view their body as a collection of separate systems to be fixed by delegated medical authorities rather than as an integrated whole. They approach healthcare with a transactional mindset, preferring clear directives from doctors rather than explanations or invitations to participate. They prefer to keep their medical issues in contained boxes, viewing their physical symptoms as disconnected from their emotional lives or past experiences. This compartmentalization can be a coping strategy that helps them function from day to day, especially when dealing with chronic conditions. However, it can also prevent them from developing insight and becoming a strong self-advocate.

This pattern often emerges from past medical experiences, generational beliefs about physician authority, or simply feeling overwhelmed by health information. While outsourcing can sometimes be practical, particularly for acute care, it frequently leads to fragmented treatment plans, missed connections between seemingly unrelated symptoms, and diminished personal agency.

Stacey had been struggling with her weight since her early twenties. By age forty, she had developed type 2 diabetes, back problems, and knee pain. She had tried numerous diets without success and wanted to lose weight and reverse her diabetes. "Just tell me what to eat and what pill to take," she said during our first meeting. "I don't have time for the psychological stuff."

But Stacey didn't need another lecture on eating less and exercising more. What she needed was to explore her relationship with food, hunger, satiety, and body image. As a child, she had been bullied for her weight. Her mother had called her "chunky" when she wasn't even overweight. Beginning in high school, shame about her body led to her overeating processed food. Her mind became numb to normal cues of hunger and satiety.

My advice wasn't to diet but to get back in touch with the feelings of hunger and satiety, to feed herself on a regular schedule, and to rekindle a more nurturing relationship with her body. When she learned not to tune out her feelings and to instead listen to hunger cues, she felt better than she had ever felt while dieting. When she came in to see me six months later weighing twenty pounds less, she was shocked that she'd actually been eating more than she ever had. "Self-compassion for the win!" I smiled.

Working with Outsourcer Tendencies

- **Strengths to leverage:** Your efficiency and clear decision-making in certain healthcare contexts can be valuable.
- **Watch for blind spots:** Treating symptoms without addressing their underlying causes leads to escalating health problems and increasing dependency on medication. Viewing your body as a collection of separate systems rather than an integrated whole leads to missing critical connections among symptoms.
- **Growth opportunities:** Begin asking "why" questions about your symptoms and treatments rather than focusing exclusively on

quick solutions. Consider how various aspects of your health might connect with one another.

The doctor-patient relationship is at the core of effective healthcare. Trust happens when both parties bring self-awareness to this relationship and communicate clearly about their biases, beliefs, and emotional responses to vulnerability. This trust becomes the foundation of shared decision-making and ultimately better health outcomes.

Understanding your patient personality creates the self-awareness necessary for the next crucial step: asking for help.

Step 4:
Ask for Help

The most empowered patients I know aren't those who navigate their health journey alone but those who have learned when and how to invite others into their process—whether medical professionals, family members, or trusted friends. To be healthy is to seek support and guidance, yet asking for help remains challenging for many of us. The right help is not always available or accessible, not to mention that asking for help requires recognizing that you need it in the first place. Your patient personality often determines not just whether you seek help but what kind of help you're willing to accept and from whom. The Optimizer might resist seeking help until they've exhausted every self-improvement strategy available. The Pleaser might ask for help but then dismiss their own needs to avoid being a burden. The Internet Warrior might seek endless second opinions online rather than trusting professional guidance. The Outsourcer might want help but only in the form of quick fixes that don't require their active participation.

The thorniest questions in medicine these days are: Whom can you trust? How can you navigate the maze of specialists, alternative practitioners, health coaches, and online experts? How can you separate evidence-based guidance from marketing hype? If you don't have a doctor who can quarterback your care, learning how to coordinate your own support becomes essential.

Getting the right help begins by identifying which elements of your health ecosystem need support. As discussed, each area may require different types of assistance—medical, psychological, social-emotional, nutritional, physical—and recognizing these needs before they become crises is crucial to maintaining your health agency. Take time to identify the *type* of support you need. For example, **information support** involves getting reliable facts, explanations, or guidance, such as asking your doctor to explain test results in plain language or researching treatment options from reputable sources. You need this when you feel confused or uninformed about your health situation. **Emotional support** means having someone listen without judgment, validate your feelings, or simply be present during difficult times. This might involve, for example, asking a friend to sit with you during a scary medical procedure or joining a support group in which others understand your struggles. **Practical support** includes tangible help with daily tasks—asking family members to prepare meals for you during recovery, arranging transportation to appointments, or having someone help organize your medications. **Advocacy support** involves having someone speak up for your needs or help navigate complex systems, for example, taking a trusted person to important medical appointments to help ask questions or working with a patient navigator to understand insurance coverage. The key is to be specific about which type of support you need. Instead of saying "I need help," try "I need someone to listen while I process this diagnosis" (emotional), "I need help understanding what this treatment involves" (informational), or "I need someone to drive me to appointments this week" (practical). When people understand exactly how they can help, they're more likely to provide effective support rather than defaulting to advice giving or problem-solving when that's not what you need.

Recognizing When You Need Help

One of the most important skills in health management is recognizing when your current approach isn't sufficient and additional support is necessary. Warning signs that self-management isn't enough often manifest themselves differently across your health ecosystem. In your INFORMATICS quadrant, you might need help when you're overwhelmed by conflicting medical information, when your test results don't make sense despite research, or when you're struggling to make sense of complex treatment options. If you find yourself spending hours researching symptoms online and feeling more confused than informed, or if you're avoiding medical appointments because you don't understand what your doctors are telling you, it's time to seek clearer guidance.

Your INPUTS quadrant signals a need for support when your relationship with food, alcohol, or substances feels out of control despite your good intentions. This isn't just about addiction—though substance abuse certainly requires professional help—but includes patterns such as emotional eating that undermines your health goals, confusion about conflicting nutritional advice, and side effects from medications or supplements that you can't manage alone.

The INFRASTRUCTURE quadrant often sends clear distress signals when physical pain persists despite rest and basic self-care, when injuries don't heal as expected, or when physical limitations begin affecting your daily functioning. Many people normalize chronic pain or movement limitations, not realizing that physical therapy, pain management, or other interventions could significantly improve their quality of life.

Your INSIGHT quadrant may be the most challenging to assess objectively, since emotional and mental health struggles can affect your ability to recognize that you need help. Warning signs include persistent sleep problems, anxiety that interferes with daily activities, sadness or hopelessness that doesn't improve with time, difficulty concentrating or making decisions, or emotional responses that feel disproportionate to circumstances. Sometimes friends or family members notice these changes before you do, making their observations valuable data rather than unwelcome interference.

Barriers to Getting Help

It's appropriate to blame our broken healthcare system for most of the barriers to care. But it's important to examine other factors, too. For example, deeply ingrained societal messages about strength, independence, and personal responsibility for health outcomes can prevent the most stoic patients from seeking advice. Fear of judgment ranks among the most common barriers. Patients often describe to me how they have been shamed, even traumatized, by medical professionals. If you've felt unheard or misunderstood by providers in the past, it's natural to approach new healthcare relationships with caution. These experiences are particularly damaging when they involve sensitive issues such as mental health, sexual health, or addiction. Building trust after being hurt by a provider requires both time and finding practitioners who demonstrate genuine understanding and respect.

Financial concerns create another layer of complexity. Even with insurance, healthcare costs can be overwhelming at best, leading people to delay or avoid seeking help. This calculation becomes more complicated when considering nonmedical support such as therapy, nutritional counseling, or alternative treatments that may not be covered by insurance. Poor access to affordable, high-quality healthcare remains one the most troubling problems in America today.

Cultural and family backgrounds also shape attitudes toward help seeking. For example, some families view mental health treatment as shameful or see physical therapy as unnecessary unless someone is severely injured. One of my patients put off a much-needed hysterectomy for what she described to me as "matriarchal pressure" to suffer through the pain. Even when your preconceptions are justified, cultivating an awareness of the ways in which you may limit, censor, or judge yourself about getting the care you need can be empowering.

Navigating Care Coordination Challenges

One of the most frustrating aspects of modern healthcare is the lack of communication among different providers. You might see a primary care doctor, a specialist, a therapist, and a physical therapist, only to discover that they have different treatment recommendations or don't know about one another's involvement in your care.

Artificial intelligence and digital health technologies hold tremendous promise for transforming this fragmented landscape. I envision a future in which your primary care doctor creates a shared care plan that will be updated in real time across all your providers, in which your physical therapist's notes about movement patterns will instantly inform your primary care doctor's understanding of your chronic pain, and in which conflicting treatment recommendations will automatically trigger consultations among providers. These technological solutions could eliminate many of the care coordination burdens that currently fall on patients and their families.

But until that technology is fully integrated into healthcare systems—and until you have access to a primary care medical "home"—learning to coordinate your own care is essential. Start by maintaining your own comprehensive health record that travels with you between providers. This includes your four-quadrant analysis, your current concerns, and your treatment goals. When providers understand your complete health picture rather than just their specialty area, they can make better recommendations and coordinate more effectively with your other providers.

Actively facilitate communication between your providers when needed. If your therapist recommends stress management techniques that might affect your blood pressure medication, make sure your primary care doctor knows about the recommendation. If your physical therapist identifies movement patterns that might relate to your chronic headaches, share this information with your neurologist. Don't assume that providers will communicate with one another automatically; often they won't unless you specifically request it.

When different providers give you conflicting advice, resist the temptation to simply choose the recommendation you prefer. Instead, bring the conflict back to both providers and ask them to clarify their reasoning. Often such conflicts arise from incomplete information rather than genuine disagreement about treatment. Sometimes one provider has information the other lacks, or they're prioritizing different aspects of your health. Understanding their reasoning will help you make informed decisions rather than choosing arbitrarily.

Set clear expectations about communication and coordination from the beginning of any provider relationship. Ask how (and if) the provider will communicate with other members of your healthcare team to coordinate care. Providers who seem reluctant to collaborate or who dismiss the importance of your other healthcare relationships may not be a good fit for comprehensive care.

Some situations require professional care coordination that even the most skilled primary care doctor cannot manage alone. If you're juggling multiple complex conditions, if you're receiving conflicting advice from several specialists, or if your health needs exceed your ability to coordinate them yourself, consider hiring a professional care managers or care navigation service.

No one achieves health in isolation. The goal isn't to become dependent on others for your health decisions; it's to build a network to support *you* and all four of your health quadrants.

Recognizing When You Need *Different* or *Better* Help

One of the most challenging aspects of being an empowered patient is recognizing when the help you're getting isn't the help you need. This isn't about being difficult or mistrustful; it's about developing discernment. Your body is giving you feedback. The question is: Are you listening to it, and are your providers listening to it?

Learning to identify red flags in your care isn't about becoming paranoid or questioning every medical recommendation. It's about recognizing patterns that suggest you need to seek different expertise, ask harder questions, or find providers who can see your complete picture. Here are warning signs that the help you're currently receiving may not be adequate, and that it's time to seek a second opinion, a different approach, or a more comprehensive evaluation.

Red Flags: When to Question Your Diagnosis and Treatment Plan

Sometimes the standard medical approach misses the mark, leading to treatments that don't address the real problem. Here are warning signs that you may need a second opinion or different approach.

Tests and Symptoms Don't Align

- Your symptoms are severe, but tests come back normal.
- Multiple tests have been ordered but have provided no actionable information.
- Different specialists interpret the same results differently.
- Each specialist focuses only on their domain without considering connections.
- No one is coordinating your care or seeing your complete picture.

Treatments Aren't Working

- You're told "This should work," but it doesn't.
- Treatments help initially but their effects diminish quickly.
- Side effects create new problems without solving the original issue.
- You've tried multiple approaches in the same category with no improvement.

Communication Red Flags

- You're told symptoms are "just stress" or "just aging" without thorough evaluation.
- You're told to "learn to live with it" without exploring all options.
- Questions about your concerns or alternative approaches are discouraged.
- Providers seem rushed and don't listen to your full story.

When These Red Flags Appear

- Seek providers who listen and assess your complete health ecosystem, not just individual symptoms.
- Consider direct primary care for a more patient-centered, holistic approach.
- Request a comprehensive review of all your symptoms together.
- Ask for second opinions, especially before surgery or starting long-term medications.
- Don't accept "normal" test results if you're still suffering.
- Document your symptoms and their patterns systematically.

Remember: You know your body better than anyone else can. If something doesn't feel right about your diagnosis or treatment plan, trust that instinct and seek additional perspectives. Advocating for yourself isn't about being difficult, it's about ensuring you receive the thorough, thoughtful care you deserve.

Recognizing these red flags is part of asking for help effectively. But knowing when to push for better answers and when to accept uncertainty leads us to perhaps the hardest step of all: practicing acceptance.

Step 5: Practice Acceptance

After you've sought appropriate help, asked the right questions, found providers who truly listen, and exhausted reasonable options—that's when acceptance becomes not resignation, but wisdom. That's when you shift from "I need different help" to "I need to work with what is." Yet arguably the most challenging aspect of being human is accepting the things we cannot control. Risk is everywhere. We face the potential for harm every time we drive a car, swallow a medication, or engage in a new relationship. To be human is to accept certain risks, including the risk of mortality.

The approach I take with patients who are facing difficult news or reckoning with uncertainty boils down to a secular version of the Serenity Prayer. We need "the serenity to accept the things [we] cannot change, courage to change the things [we] can, and the wisdom to know the difference." Whether you're an atheist, a devout Catholic, a lapsed Protestant, a Buddhist, an Orthodox Jew, a Muslim, or something else entirely, the Serenity Prayer is for you. It's a simple reminder to focus on what can be changed and to practice acceptance of things beyond your control.

Psychologists have long understood that our perception of whether we control our fate or current life situation or are at the mercy of outside events affects our health. Having the sense of taking charge of our own lives again as opposed to feeling at the mercy of outside events can restore our sense of agency and self-determination. Having a chronic disease can seem grossly unfair, yet it is something we have to endure. To do so, we can make an effort to meet ourselves where we are.

Let me be clear: Acceptance is not about agreeing with or surrendering to suffering. It is not about reckless abandonment of caution or carelessness about health. It is not about giving up. Rather, acceptance means letting go of the false promise of a risk-free medical decision. It requires ceding control where control isn't possible.

Acceptance doesn't happen in a single moment; it is a complex psychological process that unfolds over time. Understanding the process can help you navigate your journey toward accepting health challenges, limitations, or difficult decisions.

Honestly Recognizing What Is

The first step in acceptance is honestly recognizing what is. This means acknowledging difficult realities without minimizing, avoiding, or distorting them. For health issues, this might mean recognizing a chronic condition, genetic predisposition, or physical limitation. This stage often involves grief work.

When faced with health challenges, many people move through stages similar to those described in Elisabeth Kübler-Ross's five stages of grief model: denial, anger, bargaining, depression, and eventually acceptance. These aren't strict sequential stages; people often cycle through them or revisit earlier stages, as my patient Marcus did when he was diagnosed with Parkinson's disease. His initial response was denial; he attributed his tremor to stress and refused to discuss his treatment options. As the truth of the disease became undeniable, he moved through anger ("Why me?"), bargaining ("If I exercise more, maybe it will go away"), and depression as he contemplated the future. Acceptance came not as resignation but as a shift in perspective: "This is my reality. How can I live the fullest life possible within these new parameters?"

Letting Go of Resistance

The core psychological shift in acceptance involves releasing the struggle against what cannot be changed. This doesn't mean giving up but rather stopping the exhausting fight against reality. As the psychologist Carl Rogers noted, "The curious paradox is that when I accept myself just as I am, then I can change." This paradox is central to acceptance; it's only by first acknowledging your current reality that you can create space for meaningful growth.

My patient Hariette spent years fighting her diagnosis of rheumatoid arthritis. She exhausted herself trying every unproven treatment she could find, refusing to accommodate her daily life to her condition. The turning point came when she finally acknowledged that her disease was part of her life, not something she could overcome through willpower. Paradoxically, that acceptance freed her to focus her energy on evidence-based treatments and lifestyle modifications that actually improved her symptoms.

Cognitive Restructuring

Acceptance often requires reframing unhelpful thought patterns, moving from "Why me?" to "This is what is." You might shift from "I can't stand this" to "This is difficult, but I can handle it." Cognitive therapies specifically target these thought patterns, helping to distinguish between unhelpful rumination and productive problem-solving.

When my patient Marguerite was in treatment for aggressive colon cancer, she started defining herself by what she could no longer do. Her thoughts were dominated by comparisons to her previous capacities and grievances about her limitations. Through cognitive work, she gradually shifted to asking different questions. Instead of "Why can I no longer hike without feeling exhausted?" she started asking herself, "What forms of movement bring me joy now?" Instead of "How can I get my old life back?" she asked, "How can I create meaning and purpose within my new reality?"

Practicing Self-Compassion

Research shows that treating yourself with the same kindness you would offer a friend creates psychological resilience that helps navigate difficult circumstances. This means speaking to yourself kindly about your limitations, recognizing that imperfection is part of the shared human experience, and being mindful of painful feelings without suppressing or exaggerating them.

My patient Kent initially responded to his diagnosis of diabetes with harsh self-criticism. Feelings of shame and self-loathing led to more problematic eating, creating a destructive cycle. Learning self-compassion with the help of his rabbi helped transform his relationship with his condition. He learned to give himself permission to be human, to have a difficult day, but not to let it define him or dictate his choices for the next day.

Aligning with Your Values

Acceptance is most powerful when coupled with value-directed behavior. This means identifying what truly matters to you and taking action in those directions, even with limitations present. For example, someone with chronic pain might accept their condition while simultaneously committing to maintaining meaningful relationships, pursuing modified versions of activities they love, or finding new paths to purpose.

Therapeutic Approaches That Foster Acceptance

Several evidence-based therapies can help when you're struggling to accept things beyond your control.

Acceptance and commitment therapy (ACT) focuses on psychological flexibility through embracing thoughts and feelings without trying to change them and practicing nonjudgmental awareness of the "here and now." Rather than trying to eliminate difficult feelings, ACT helps people make room for them while building a meaningful life.

Dialectical behavioral therapy (DBT) teaches acceptance skills including mindfulness (observing without judgment), distress tolerance (surviving crises without making things worse), and radical acceptance (completely accepting reality as it is). DBT shows that you can accept yourself completely while working toward change.

Mindfulness-based approaches train your attention to stay with present-moment experience without judgment. Regular meditation practice helps develop the capacity to observe difficult thoughts and sensations without immediately reacting to them. My patient Patricia found that mindfulness meditation gave her a new relationship with her chronic pain symptoms. Before training in meditation, she was constantly fighting the pain and tightening her body around it, which only made it worse. Through mindfulness, she learned to observe the pain without adding layers of resistance and frustration. The pain was still there, but it no longer controlled her life.

Additionally, **psychotherapy** and **grief counseling** can provide crucial support during the acceptance process. Spiritual guidance often helps people find meaning within suffering. The research on psilocybin-assisted therapy shows promise for helping people with terminal diagnoses work through existential anxiety and find peace with mortality. This treatment remains investigational only and is not yet widely available; however, I hope it gains FDA approval in my lifetime.

When Acceptance Becomes Essential: Facing Your Mortality

My patient Nora had been living with metastatic breast cancer for four years, and her CT scan showed that it was spreading deeper into her body. Every time she asked her oncologist about her prognosis, he said she needed to stay positive and keep fighting. But she felt terrible most days due to bone pain and weakness. She wanted to attend her daughter's wedding, planned for the following spring, but she also didn't want to spend whatever time she had left feeling so sick.

Nora's story isn't unique. She represents thousands of patients caught in a healthcare system that has forgotten how to talk honestly about dying. Her oncologist, well-meaning and skilled, was treating her cancer but not *her*. I understand why this happens. Doctors are trained to see a problem and fix it. We aren't as adept at sitting with uncertainty, witnessing suffering, and having hard conversations about things we cannot control. But we have to.

One of the hardest things I do as a doctor is tell people truths they don't want to hear. But I've learned that honesty, delivered with compassion, is often the greatest gift we can give. Nora needed to understand that her cancer was not going to be cured. That didn't mean there was nothing we could do; it meant we needed to shift our focus from trying to eliminate the cancer to optimizing her quality of life with the cancer. It meant accepting that death was near.

I explained the risks and limitations of further chemotherapy. I explained that opting for comfort care instead wasn't about "giving up"; it meant choosing to fight for different things: peace, connection, dignity, and time that felt meaningful rather than just medical. The conversation was difficult, but sometimes the most healing thing we can do is witness someone's pain without trying to fix it away.

I didn't start by talking about Nora's treatment options. I started by asking her what was most important to her right now. What did she want the next few months to look like? What would make her feel as though she was living, not just surviving? She wanted to have energy to talk with her daughter about the wedding and marriage. She wanted to travel to see her sister one more time. She wanted to feel like herself when she looked in the mirror. She wanted to be mentally sharp enough to finish writing letters to her five best friends. Those weren't medical goals, they were life goals. And they had everything to do with her medical decisions.

When we looked at the chemotherapy protocol her oncologist had recommended through that lens, the choice became clearer. The treatment had a small chance of extending her life by a few months but a high likelihood of causing fatigue, nausea, and cognitive fog that would interfere with everything she'd just told me mattered most.

After our conversation, Nora decided to stop chemotherapy and enroll in hospice care. It wasn't a decision born from despair; it was a decision born from clarity about her values and priorities. Acceptance of her situation wasn't about giving up hope; it was about hoping for different things: comfort instead of cure, quality instead of quantity, presence instead of procedures. She wanted to have meaningful time with her family, peaceful moments, the chance to say the things that mattered.

She lived for four more months. She attended her daughter's wedding. She took the trip to see her sister. She finished the letters to her friends. She died at home, not because home death is inherently better but because that was what she and her family chose when given options and honest dialogue.

You don't have to be facing a terminal diagnosis to benefit from thinking about these questions. In fact, it's better if you consider them while you're healthy and not in crisis. Start by reflecting on what gives your life meaning. What quality-of-life factors, if lost, would be unacceptable to you? Have conversations with the people you love about what matters most to you. These shouldn't be onetime discussions but ongoing conversations that will evolve as your life and health change.

Nora's story isn't ultimately about dying; it's about living. It's about making conscious choices aligned with your values instead of defaulting to whatever the medical system offers. It's about recognizing that sometimes the most loving thing we can do is let go. It's about understanding that dignity isn't about the setting or circumstances of our death but about whether we feel honored as whole human beings.

Perhaps most important, acceptance isn't a destination you reach once and inhabit forever. Like physical fitness or emotional intelligence, it's a skill that requires ongoing practice and regular renewal. My patient David, living with Parkinson's disease for over a decade, describes it this way: "Some days I wake up and have to accept all over again that my body doesn't work the way it used to. But I've gotten better at it. The path back to acceptance gets shorter each time I practice it."

The good news is that like any other skill, acceptance becomes easier with practice. The neural pathways associated with acceptance strengthen over time, allowing more flexibility and resilience in facing life's inevitable challenges. Learning to make peace with uncertainty—to make the best decisions possible with the information available while accepting that complete certainty is unattainable—is a crucial step toward establishing health agency. It allows you to move forward with thoughtful choices rather than remaining paralyzed by the search for perfect answers. In this way, acceptance becomes its own form of empowerment. By accepting what you cannot change, you free up precious energy and attention for the areas in which your actions can make a real difference.

Remember that acceptance, like all other aspects of health, is a practice rather than a destination—something to be cultivated with patience, compassion, and ongoing attention. The goal isn't to become someone who never struggles with difficult realities but someone who can move through that struggle more skillfully, with greater self-compassion, and with a clearer focus on what truly matters.

The Three A's: Your Foundation of Health Agency

Throughout this book, we've explored a framework to reclaim your health. This journey culminates in what I call the Three A's—the foundation of true health agency:

Awareness

The first A is awareness about your health ecosystem and how its parts interrelate. This means understanding your medical data, your inputs, your physical infrastructure, and your mental and emotional patterns. It means recognizing how each of these domains affects the others, creating a complex web of influences on your overall well-being. Awareness is about seeing clearly, without distortion or denial, the reality of your current health situation.

Acceptance

The second A is acceptance of the elements of your health ecosystem that you cannot control—genetic predispositions, past traumas, chronic conditions, or life circumstances that simply are. Acceptance doesn't mean liking these realities or believing that they're fair. It means acknowledging them as part of your current landscape so you can work with them rather than exhausting yourself fighting against them.

Agency

The third A is agency—taking informed, intentional action in the domains where you can make a difference. Agency emerges naturally from the foundation of awareness and acceptance. When you clearly see your health reality and accept what cannot be changed, you can direct your energy toward what can be influenced.

These three A's work together synergistically. You might have to accept a genetic predisposition to diabetes, but you can transform your relationship with food and work with your doctor to consider new treatments such as GLP-1 medications to lose weight. If you have menopausal symptoms, you can decide for yourself whether the benefits of hormone replacement therapy outweigh the risks in your individual situation, then sleep well knowing you made the best decision possible based on the information available.

KNOW YOURSELF, ADVOCATE FOR YOURSELF

Putting It All Together
Self-Reflection and Action Guide

PART 1 Self-Reflection: Owning Your Role in Your Own Healthcare

Now let's consider how to operationalize your four-quadrant health map—using your personal definition of health as your compass and these questions as your guide:

Seeing the Whole Picture

- When you look across all four quadrants (INFORMATICS, INPUTS, INFRASTRUCTURE, INSIGHT), what connections do you notice between them? (For example: How does stress affect what you eat? How does chronic pain affect your mood? How does your inner critic affect your everyday habits?)
- Which quadrant feels strongest for you right now? Which feels most neglected?
- If your health were a company, what would be your top three priorities as CEO?

Your Patient Personality

- When you walk into a doctor's office, what version of yourself shows up? Anxious? Apologetic? Demanding? Deferential?
- Think about your last few healthcare encounters—what went well? What didn't?
- What patient personality tendencies help you get good care? Which ones get in your way?
- Do you tend to be: The Optimizer (always trying to perfect your health)? The Pleaser (agreeing even when you shouldn't)? The Internet Warrior (researching everything obsessively)? The Outsourcer (delegating without understanding)?
- How do different providers bring out different sides of you?
- What communication strategies work best for you? What falls flat?

Asking for Help (The Practical Stuff)

- Looking at all four quadrants, where do you most need support right now?
- What's your current healthcare team? Who's missing?
- If you could design your ideal support system, what would it include? Primary care doctor? Therapist? Nutritionist? Physical therapist? Trusted friend who keeps you accountable?
- What specific barriers prevent you from asking for help? Money? Time? Pride? Fear of being dismissed? Not knowing who to ask?
- What questions have you been afraid to ask your providers? Write them down.
- Who in your life could you enlist as a health advocate—someone to come to appointments with you or help you make decisions?
- What's one concrete step you could take this week toward getting the help you need?

Acceptance (The Hardest Part)

- What aspects of your health are you still fighting against rather than working with?
- What do you wish you could change but realistically cannot? How much physical or mental energy are you spending on that wish?
- Where are you seeking certainty that doesn't exist? (Perfect test results? Guaranteed outcomes? A diagnosis that explains everything? Immortality?)
- What health issues might you be able to accept if you reframed the problem as one to manage, not "fix"?
- What would it look like to adapt to—rather than eliminate—a health challenge?
- What small act of acceptance could you practice this week? (Example: Accepting that you need eight hours of sleep, not six. Accepting that you can't eat certain foods without consequences. Accepting that your body has changed.)
- If you accepted your current limitations, what energy would be freed up for actually improving what CAN be changed?

Your Action Plan

- What's one small change in each quadrant you could make this week? This year?
- What do you need to say NO to in order to prioritize your health?
- Who will hold you accountable?
- How will you measure success? What will you do to celebrate wins?

PART 2 Healthcare Conversations: Questions and Strategies for Medical Encounters

Questions to Ask Your Medical Provider

- "I'm trying to take a more comprehensive approach to my health. Based on what you know about me, who else should I have on my team?"
- "Is there anything I can do on my end to better communicate to you and other medical professionals about my health issues?"
- "What would you say or recommend to me if you weren't afraid of worrying me or hurting my feelings?"
- "Can you help me understand when I should handle something on my own versus when I need to bring in a specialist?"
- "I'm getting conflicting advice from different providers. Can you help me sort through it?"
- "I'm having trouble accepting that [this condition/limitation/diagnosis] might be permanent. How have your other patients dealt with this?"
- "What can I realistically improve versus what do I need to learn to live with?"
- "What quality-of-life improvements are possible, even if there is no cure?"
- "How should we measure success beyond just the numbers or test results?"

Communication Strategies

- Write down your three most important concerns before the appointment.
- Bring someone with you to important appointments.

- Keep a one-page health summary with your current conditions, medications, and recent test results.
- After appointments, send your provider a message summarizing what you understood and asking them to correct anything you got wrong.
- When you don't understand something, say: "I want to make sure I can explain this to my [partner/family]. Can you say that another way?"
- Frame discussions around your quality-of-life and functional goals rather than just symptom elimination.
- Bring clear examples of activities or functions that matter most to you to help focus treatment priorities.

The Last Word: The Empowered Patient as a Catalyst for Change

You've now traveled through your complete health ecosystem: mapping your INFORMATICS, taking conscious control of your INPUTS, understanding your INFRASTRUCTURE, and exploring your INSIGHT. You are armed with a map of your four quadrants, the language to navigate medical complexity, and permission to ask for what you need.

The next question is: What will you do with this knowledge?

Start with yourself. Use the "Know Yourself, Advocate for Yourself" reflection and action guides woven throughout this book. Notice the connections among your quadrants that you may never have recognized before. Practice the five steps: Redefine health on your own terms, understand your unique ecosystem, recognize your patient personality, learn to ask for help effectively, and practice acceptance of what cannot be changed while focusing your energy on what you can influence.

Then refuse to accept the status quo. When healthcare providers rush through appointments without understanding your complete story, speak up. When systems treat you like a collection of symptoms rather than a whole human being, advocate for being recognized as a person not a diagnosis. Changing our healthcare system will require empowered patients who understand what healthcare looks like and refuse to accept anything less. It will require individuals who see their own health journey as connected to broader questions of justice, access, and human dignity.

Extend your influence. Share what you've learned with family members who might benefit from this approach. Advocate for the kind of healthcare you and your loved ones deserve. Support policies and providers that prioritize comprehensive, relationship-centered care. Use your voice and your vote to demand that primary care become accessible to all Americans, not just those privileged enough to afford it.

By inviting the mess of being human into your healthcare conversation, you acknowledge that bodies aren't machines to be optimized but complex ecosystems to be understood. When you learn to articulate how your stress affects your sleep and how your sleep impacts your eating patterns, you've discovered what millions of Americans need to understand: that health isn't about having all the answers, it's about asking better questions.

You don't need to become a healthcare activist or take responsibility for fixing our broken system. You just need to own your health story and model self-advocacy and care. Start small and dream big. This work is messy and deeply personal. It requires access to the truth and the courage to face it. It demands scientific accuracy and compassionate flexibility. It requires finding trusted guides and relinquishing control, over and over again. There's no trophy for suffering in silence, no medal for avoiding difficult conversations, and certainly no health benefit to pretending you've got it all figured out.

Sometimes the bravest health decision is saying "I need help" or "This is where I am right now." Your health story is written not in permanent ink but in pencil with a fresh eraser. The framework you've learned provides the structure, but you provide the content. The quadrants provide the map, but you choose the destination.

Focus on your four quadrants. Practice the five steps. Become the kind of patient you'd want your loved ones to be. The broader change is already happening, one empowered patient at a time.

The next chapter is waiting for you to write it. Make it a good one.

Acknowledgments

This book would not exist without the extraordinary support of many people.

To my editor, Lauren Marino, and the entire team at Simon & Schuster: Thank you for believing in this project and for your patience, guidance, and expertise in bringing it to life. Lauren, I knew you were the right woman for the job the first time I met you, crowded into a New York City restaurant booth together, drinking cocktails and sharing our life stories. Thank you for your insight and direction and for pushing me beyond what I thought was possible.

To Lyric Winik, my writing coach: Thank you for helping me find my voice and for teaching me how to translate my experience of patient care into words on the page. You treat the written word like you do the people around you—with care and nurture. Your dry sense of humor and your humanity kept me sane during the writing process. Thank you for your wisdom and steadfast guidance that brought this book to life.

To my dear friends who have supported and humored me throughout this process: Thank you for listening to me talk endlessly about this book, for your encouragement when I doubted myself, and for reminding me why this work matters. Your friendship sustains me.

To my patients: The stories in this book are inspired by the resilience and wisdom you demonstrate every day. Thank you for trusting me with your care and for teaching me what it truly means to heal. This book is for you and because of you.

To my parents, my brother Walter, and the entire Martin-Leithauser-McBride crew: Your love and support are my foundation. I am the luckiest person alive to be part of our family. Thank you for having my back in good times and bad.

To my brother Harry: Your tender heart, your unwavering humor, and your courageous fight to get better taught me more about resilience than anything I learned in medical school. I carry your spirit with me everywhere.

And finally, to my children, Henry, George, and Stella: You are my greatest teachers in courage and kindness, levity and humility. Thank you for reminding me every day what matters most.

Index

R

S

T

X

Y

Z

About the Author

DR. LUCY McBRIDE is a primary care physician and cofounder of the Ackerly McBride Group in Washington, DC, where she has been caring for patients for over twenty-five years. A graduate of Princeton University and Harvard Medical School, with a master's degree in pharmacology from the University of Cambridge as a Fulbright Scholar, she completed her medical training at Johns Hopkins Hospital.

During the COVID-19 pandemic, Dr. McBride became a nationally recognized voice on the importance of addressing mental and physical health in tandem. She is the author of the popular weekly medical newsletter *Are You Okay?* and hosts the podcast *Beyond the Prescription,* where she pulls back the curtain on what it means to be healthy.

Her writing has been published in *The Atlantic*, *The Washington Post*, and *USA Today*, and she has appeared on CNN, MSNBC, NPR, and PBS, advocating for a data-driven, patient-centered, holistic approach to healthcare.

Dr. McBride believes that health is more than the absence of disease—it's about awareness of our medical facts, acceptance of the things we cannot control, and agency over what we can change. Health, she argues, is a process, not an outcome. Known for her compassionate approach and ability to distill complex medical topics into accessible conversations, Dr. McBride empowers patients with evidence-based information and nuanced guidance for everyday health decisions.

A native Washingtonian, she lives in DC with her husband, two blocks from her parents. She is the proud mother of three grown children. You can find her work at LucyMcBride.com.